QI GONG

QI GONG
Rediscovering
Our Humanity

Paul Fraser

AEON

First published in 2019 by
Aeon Books Ltd
12 New College Parade
Finchley Road
London NW3 5EP

British Library Cataloguing in Publication Data

A C.I.P. for this book is available from the British Library

ISBN-13: 978-1-91280-706-2

Typeset by Medlar Publishing Solutions Pvt Ltd, India
Printed in Great Britain

www.aeonbooks.co.uk

For
Anisha,
A True Partner in Love, Life
and
This Path We Share

Contents

Acknowledgements

The help, guidance, and encouragement I've received has been much and from many people. I would like to mention a few of them here, knowing that the depth of my gratitude is beyond any words I can find.

Master Ou, Wen Wei. The best teacher and example I have ever had.

Mandy Ou for treating us all like family and being a mother to us all.

Olivia Ou for tirelessly arranging events and acting as an interpreter, facilitator and good friend.

Sing Yu for your friendship, great example, and photography skills.

Adam Sommer of the "Holes to Heavens" podcast, gifted astrologer, good friend, and the catalyst for this book.

Tom Tam, for saving my life, being my first teacher, and introducing me to a world I had no idea existed.

Master Vincent (Fong) Chu of the Gin Soon Tai Chi Federation, whose Tai Qi skills are only matched by his generosity in teaching.

Sifu Dimitri Mougdis of The Internal Arts Institute of Stuart, Florida, a brilliant Tai Qi instructor with tremendous warmth and humor.

Closer to home: My wife, Anisha Desai Fraser for your love, patience, and thoughtful feedback, and our dog, Jade, great sage of unconditional love.

Preface

"[C]oincidence exists in necessity. Without necessity, no coincidence. How could necessity come into being if there were no coincidence? Many coincidences make a necessity."
—*The Path of Life, Vol. III*, Translated English Edition 2003
Ou, Wen Wei, Qigong Master

I dismissed those words at first; I found them confusing. Later, I tried to make sense of them, eventually coming to the realization that every pivotal moment I could recall came about through coincidence. It seemed as if there had been some guiding force that appeared, random in the moment, but, in hindsight, fitting a discernible pattern.

As human beings I suppose most of us strive to make meaning from the events of our lives. It is understandable. Our lives are all we have. They are important to us. Why would we not seek to make what occurs within them matter? In the end it may make no difference if there is a guiding presence or not, as long as we value what we do and do what we value.

Looking back, I may have been one of the least likely candidates for exploring the art and science of qigong. Everything about my knowledge and experience was conventional and, at best, average. But then a very unconventional illness presented itself and the average avenues of treatment were not enough. Through a series of coincidences, I found myself at first helped and then later transformed by qigong.

Adding to those coincidences, the place I lived at the time, Boston, Massachusetts, was home to tremendous talent when it came to qigong. There was Tom Tam, my first teacher and the man I credit with saving my life; Dr. Yang, Jwing-Ming of Yang's Martial Arts Association, scholar and author of numerous books on the subject; Master Vincent (Fong) Chu of the Gin Soon Tai Chi Federation; Lin, Soong of the Lin family (Wild Goose Qigong), famous for generations as qigong practitioners, who once, using only qi, repositioned a herniated disc in my lumbar; and Daoist Priest Zhou, Xuan-Yun, who grew up on Wudang Mountain mastering medicine, all of the Wudang martial systems, and Daoist ritual—just to name a few. I found myself in great need and encountered much greater talent and ability.

In another work, *Pangu Mystical Qigong*, Master Ou describes the purpose of human evolution as harmony of heaven, earth and humanity. We are part of a vast network of Life, bridged by qi and spirit. Tracking our evolution may be viewed through three key stages: "[material, circumstances and people are] coexisting relatively [antagonistic], tolerating each other then becoming stable, being harmonious then resonant."

My study of qigong followed this pattern. I went from illness (coexisting antagonism), to learning, practice and health (tolerance and stability) and on to endless fascination (harmonious and resonant). In the process I found a way of living that continues to offer value and meaning, made the best friends anyone could hope for, experienced deep love in many forms, and have known the incomparable joy of helping others.

The debt I feel I owe to my teachers, to those who kept this priceless body of knowledge alive, is, I'm afraid, well beyond my capacity to repay, despite their insistence that there is no such debt. I have their examples of hard work, generosity and kindness. They make me want to try, despite myself, to offer just a fraction of what they give, hoping, in some way, to honor those gifts.

Paul Fraser
Asheville, North Carolina, USA

Introduction

Initiations

"It was involuntary. They sank my boat."

— John F. Kennedy

Like many nineteen year-olds, I had a vision of how my life would unfold. At the time, mine had something to do with investment banking, homes throughout the world, and, in later years, a Pulitzer Prize.

That vision changed abruptly, coming from another vision in a hospital bed.

Six years earlier, at thirteen, I had a respiratory illness that developed into pneumonia. In the course of a chest x-ray a strange shadow was, quite by accident, seen by a passing orthopedic surgeon as anomalies in parts of my skeleton. He mentioned it to the radiologist, who reported it to my pediatrician, who then consulted with that same orthopedic surgeon.

It was an extremely rare bone disease. It was a type of growth that infiltrated the bones on either the right or left side of the body. Generally it was nothing to worry about, and would remain for one's entire life undetected, but, in my case, it was strangely active. It had all but destroyed a section of my right humerus (the upper arm). A fall, or even excessive pressure would most likely result in a break. Further scans noted similar growths of a more benign nature in my ribs, two fingers, and the right side of my pelvis. Surgery was scheduled within the next couple of months and my right humerus was reconstructed with bone taken from my left hip. After physical therapy I was cleared to resume my normal, awkward teenage years. I would, however, need to have the growths in the ribs, fingers, and pelvis checked every six months or so. Once I stopped growing there would no further need for concern.

I began university studies at eighteen. All seemed well as I took on the full course load of a Finance major, made new friends, took up intramural martial arts, and explored the many diversions Boston had to offer. In the middle of my sophomore year it was time for another bone scan, most likely to be my last since I had stopped growing, this time using what was then the relatively new technology of Magnetic Resonance Imaging. The results had always shown no change in activity of the growths; there was no reason to suspect anything else.

The results of what was to be my last scan were very different and very unusual. The growth in the pelvis had become so active that much of my iliac crest was affected. The change had been so dramatic over the past six months it was very possible the growth had become malignant. Immediate surgery was scheduled to remove the growth, have it biopsied, and repair the pelvis with another bone graft.

That surgery was much longer and more involved than the previous one. When I awoke from the anesthesia there was a great deal more pain. I was grateful for the morphine and became acutely aware of its absence every four hours. When the surgeon told me that the biopsy showed cancer activity, the fear, pain, and opiate effects of the morphine mixed together, producing a kind of vague, disbelieving disassociation. We would talk about it later, he said, perhaps after my family arrived and I was feeling a little stronger.

There wasn't much more to say, it turned out. The tumor, about the size of a softball, had been removed. It was such a rare disease that no blood tests had yet been developed to track its activity. All we could do was continue to watch and wait. And hope.

I lay there with my right leg attached to a traction device, a drain inserted into the incision to remove debris from the surgery, with uneaten green jello on a nearby tray, staring at the ceiling, trying not to worry, counting the minutes to the next morphine injection, as the pain ebbed its way back. There was a crash of metal on floor as something was dropped outside my hospital room. The vibration from the crash sent new waves of pain through my pelvis. I closed my eyes and exhaled. My heart was beating fast, from pain, being startled, and worry that my life could end much sooner than I expected. I glanced at the clock. Twenty minutes to go until morphine.

It wasn't sleep but I felt strangely relaxed and heavy. My heart slowed, my breathing evened out as the pain seemed to lessen with each exhalation. Behind my eyelids images of tiny squares covered my field of vision. Gradually the squares formed an intricate pattern of what appeared to be colorful tiles—a mosaic. I could no longer feel any specific part of my body, only a sense of one part of me sinking heavily and another floating lightly, gazing down at the mosaic.

The field of vision closed in to a small grouping of colorful tiles, different shades of sky blue and cloud white. My attention went to one blue tile in particular. It seemed to become brighter, outlined with a light shimmer of gold light. A hand appeared and pointed to the tile. There were no audible words, just a strong sense of "this tile is you."

The visual field broadened, showing several hundred surrounding tiles. Two fingers of the hand plucked the tile that was me from the mosaic. As the tile was plucked, about two thirds of the surrounding tiles fell away. The tile was placed back. All the tiles that had fallen away repositioned themselves in their original places, with the entire section of the mosaic outlined in that same golden shimmer of light. "This is why you won't die," I felt. With that, a strong wave-like feeling passed through my body and I was abruptly awake.

But different.

The first noticeable sensation was actually the absence of one: I felt no pain. I was calm, happy, with a sense of eagerly anticipating some stroke of good fortune. The hospital room was the same, yet I sensed a vibrancy to my surroundings I'd never experienced before.

A nurse walked in and smiled, asking if I was ready for a dose of morphine. "No, thank you," I said, "I feel fine. I'll wait for a while until I really need it." Was I sure? I was. Did I know it was always a good idea to be medicated ahead of the pain, that it was the best way to keep it managed? I did. I remembered us talking about that. "Thank you for caring so much." I felt tears come to my eyes. I could feel something about her. She had genuine compassion. It made her happy to take care of people. She had always been like that since she could remember. How did I know that? *Did* I know that? Was I just creating a story?

Hours passed. I didn't surf through television channels, try to read anything or have any desire to direct my attention to anything other than my own sense of being. It was comfortable and interesting just *being*. I was pleasantly surprised. I had never felt like that before. I had always needed some way of occupying myself, even when I ate: I wanted something to read, to watch, someone to talk with.

I was offered more pain medication. I would need it, she said. Later in the day she would try to stand me up, perhaps take a few steps or even try some crutches. These actions were often painful, at first, right after surgery. That sounded great. I was ready. I wouldn't need the medication. I was doing well without it. Was I being honest with her and, more importantly, with myself? I was. She sighed. "All right," she said dubiously, "we'll try."

Standing and walking with crutches wasn't nearly as problematic as the group of one doctor, a physical therapist, and two nurses, all waiting to catch me, seemed to suggest. I moved down the hallway. "Practicing," I said, to kind admonishment. I ought not to rush things, they told me, and I certainly should not fall.

After two days I was left to my own devices. I could get up and roam the halls on crutches whenever I liked. I passed one of the other hospital rooms. It was filled with people, family for a woman who had been severely injured somehow. She was in a large traction device that held most of her body in place and rotated, automatically, on an even larger wheel, periodically. There was a small girl in the room, perhaps five or six years old. Her daughter. No one seemed to be paying attention to her. She was very frightened. She stepped out of the room and sat down on the floor in the hallway with silent tears streaming down her face. We looked at each other. I could feel her being afraid, sad, her love for her mother, her confusion, her desire to be both close to her mother and far, very far, from this place. It rushed through me and, for a split second, I was sure I would break the rule of not falling. I offered what I am sure was a weak smile. She smiled back, then was led back into the room by someone who had realized she wasn't there.

I returned to my room and cried.

Two more days passed and the feeling of being deeply connected with people, places, circumstances and with myself was gradually slipping away. I felt panic. I tried to hold onto the connected feeling, but the more I tried the more quickly it would dissipate. In its place I could feel worry, uncertainty, and more anxiety than before. The pain returned and, once again, I happily accepted medication.

I was sent home with detailed instructions for my own rehabilitation. I was young and this wouldn't be a problem. I would regain my strength in no time. After all, look how well I had been doing.

Except that I wasn't doing well. My blood pressure shot up to a level that was considered just below dangerous. Whenever I ate I had difficulty keeping the food down. I wasn't sleeping, was anxious almost constantly. With post-operative check-ups it was determined that the bone was not filling in the pelvis. I wasn't healing. The physicians, my family, and a few friends were sure this was some kind of post-traumatic stress. I should talk with someone; a therapist or perhaps a priest.

I was sure that talking wouldn't help. The sensations, even the anxiety, felt more in my body than my mind. Besides, I thought, how could I explain my experiences in the hospital? Would anyone believe or understand? For all the good people I had in my life, the mystical wasn't something they were likely to embrace. It wasn't how we lived.

I went to a library and searched for books related to mystical experiences. All I could find (this was 1987, after all) were books that described visions and occurrences that were far more elaborate and long-lasting than mine.

My physical condition was going from bad to worse. I was rapidly losing weight, signs of sleep deprivation were clearly apparent, my blood pressure stayed high enough that there was talk of medication, and the condition of the pelvis was unchanged. I felt very weak and was sure I was dying. I began avoiding family and friends, unable to meet worried looks and offers of advice I could not take.

On my way to yet another library, I stood, supported by crutches, on the subway platform at Wollaston station. Idly I glanced up, and saw a sign that was written half in English and half in Chinese characters: *Lea Tam Acupuncture Center*. After the words passed through my mind I felt the same wave-like sensation that brought me out of my reverie in the hospital. Suddenly, I felt infused with a sense of calm and confidence. The train came and went as I stood there staring at the sign, afraid to move, thinking that, if I did, this blissful feeling would be gone.

Twenty minutes passed as I stood, unmoving.

To hell with it. I'm going over there.

Tom Tam sat behind a desk in the waiting room. He greeted me and asked why I was there. I unloaded, not even thinking that English wasn't his original language, that I ought to slow down, and that he may only have been getting about every third word. I barely paused to breathe as I recounted the details of the strange illness, the more unusual occurrence of it becoming malignant, the downward spiral I was experiencing post-surgery, culminating with one question: Can you help me?

He smiled and answered, "Yes". How could he be so sure? I blurted. "It's my job to know," he explained, "and anyway, I can treat you and, if you don't feel better, don't pay me."

Well, there's confidence, for you, I thought, then explained that, even if I felt better, I couldn't pay him since I hadn't planned on coming in and all I was carrying were two subway tokens and a library card.

He held eye contact for a few seconds and smiled. "It's OK. You'll come back. You keep your word. Now, would you like to try acupuncture?"

I would. And did. He helped me onto a treatment table and inserted the needles in my back, legs, and arms. After asking if I was OK so far, he made circular motions with his hands over the needles. The wave-like sensations began again. I drifted into a state that was neither asleep nor awake. I could feel tension, pain, stomach discomfort, pressure in my head I hadn't noticed before: all seemed to lift to the surface and be carried away down my back, through my legs, and out of my body. I fell asleep.

I awoke to Tom removing the needles and asking me how I was doing. I looked at the clock. It had been thirty-five minutes since I got onto the table. He helped me up and I stood, unaided, feeling as if I were standing straight for the first time in about six weeks. The inside of my body felt substantial in way I had almost forgotten. After about a minute I felt my physical structure pull me down into a familiar slouch.

Tom had been watching and explained that it was a good sign. The qi—did I know what qi was? Not really? Well, the qi, or energy in my body had begun to enter the injured and imbalanced places. As it did so, I would heal much more quickly. My body couldn't yet sustain a fully upright position because my structure would need time to repair itself. The qi was already in place, which was why I felt normal for a few seconds.

May I come back tomorrow? "Best to wait a couple of days to let the qi do its work," he explained. We made another appointment and I continued on to the library and took out the only book on acupuncture I could find, reading it twice before I saw him again.

At our next meeting I showed him the book and, with a nineteen year-old's lack of humility, proceeded to explain to him what he did for a living. He smiled. Much of what was in the book was accurate, but there was a great deal that wasn't. Take, for example, causes of disease. It is much more complicated than what was explained in only a few sentences.

Tom's explanation went something like this.

Since energetic factors are key elements in our healing processes, it stands to reason that, when these factors become imbalanced, they become the causes for disease and disharmony.

Many diseases and disorders have obvious causes. Someone sneezes on you in line at the grocery store and, hours later, you have a scratchy throat. Maybe the food you had at your favorite take-out place wasn't cooked as well as it should have been and now you're experiencing gastric distress. Or perhaps you have been exposed to a harmful or toxic substance and are now experiencing signs of being poisoned. These are obvious.

But many illness are not so obvious. No one is really sure why a person's immune system doesn't identify mutated cells in his body that later become malignant and multiply into cancerous tumors, especially when this person has lived a fairly healthy and responsible lifestyle. The causes for diseases of the nervous system such as Multiple Sclerosis and Lou Gherig's Disease have baffled researchers since their discovery. Genetic research shows the presence of inherited genes that may "activate" in some people and create disease, but no one really knows why these genes activate in some people and remain dormant in others. Just as baffling is why some people never seem to get sick and others seem to contract everything.

From an energetic point of view, disease can be viewed as energy that is disharmonious to the overall health and well-being of a person. This energy can be introduced through obvious means, such as a sneeze or contaminated food. Or through more subtle ways.

Suppose you're driving to work during rush hour and it's a particularly bad day for traffic. Other motorists are just as eager, and, therefore, anxious, to get to their destinations. No one has time to spare. People are being cut off, honking, yelling, and generally behaving in ways that create distress. Once you get to work, you're already in a heightened state of anxiety, only to find out that something has gone wrong, your full workload is about to get even heavier, and everyone seems angry. You have too much to do, and so are unable to take a break. Lunch must be delivered to your desk. You eat and work. As you are eating, your stress and that of those around you becomes part of your lunch.

When your work day ends (later than usual) you go home to find that your significant other has had an equally bad day. Of course, you may not be your most balanced and understanding self; there was the horrible traffic, the greasy, undigested lunch, and long working day. Either you or your significant other says something that gets misinterpreted and perhaps an argument begins. The tension continues through dinner. Both of you may have the good sense not to argue and eat, but intuitively you know you are also absorbing the energetic circumstances of the meal.

Still, the meal isn't pleasant or relaxing, and you're thinking that you'd like to have at least one pleasant sensation today, so you have bowl of ice-cream to fill the void.

You end the day by watching television. A comedy to cheer you up. But the comedy keeps being interrupted by commercial messages that give you the unconscious impression that you won't be happy unless you spend more than you can afford on things you do not need, which may have been part of the reasoning you picked that high-stress job in the first place.

Tom paused.

When you think about disease and an unusually stressful day, how does your body feel? Pleasant or uncomfortable? The tightening in your chest and stomach are reactions to disharmonious energy. You're closing down to the flow of energy because, at the moment, the energy you're taking in isn't good for you. Now, if you replayed your stressful days, giving them focus, attention and energy, you'd be amplifying their effects. You'd be interrupting the qi-flow through your body, since you've closed down, as a defense, to what feels negative. You've absorbed harmful energy from stressful circumstances and your reactions to them. Then you've cut yourself off from the healthy flow of universal energy while trying to defend against them. Then you've amplified the disharmony within your body by giving it attention, focus, and energy.

Many people live this way for a long time and manage to stay reasonably healthy. Until they don't.

These stresses have frequencies. They can create illness in the body if amplified or left stagnant in your energetic structure. Then they accumulate.

Energy attracts similar energy. It's all magnetic. This will serve to create a disease or to activate a disease that is lying dormant. If grief sits for a long time in a body it can weaken the lungs. If similar weakening frequencies are added to that grief it can create an illness. These frequencies can be induced from substances, day-to-day stress, traumatic experiences, or they may even be passed on from parents to children, since they share an energetic structure as well as DNA. If that energy becomes so strong that it becomes a dominating force within the lungs, the cells may mutate so that they can survive in that energy. This is often the case with cancer, he explained.

Solving the problem means breaking the cycle. Strengthening qi will give you the energy to deal with stress better and will add power to immunity. It acts as insulation as it clears out disharmonies already moving through your energetic structure.

Becoming calmer, you react less. This new focus turns to that which is healthy and life-promoting. Since similar energy attracts a similar energy, you will gradually build up a strong reserve of healthy qi. Over time you'll be vital, balanced, happy, and peaceful.

It made sense. I thought for a moment, and then continued my interrogation.

What about him waving his hands over me and the sensations I felt and how quickly I felt better once he started to do that?

That was Fa Gong, emitting qi to help someone heal.

How had he done it? Can anyone learn it? Do you have to be special?

You don't have to be special, he explained, just alive. First, I would have to learn to exercise the qi to make it strong, to heal myself, to make sure that the cancer would not return. Then it would be easy enough to learn to emit qi to help other people.

So, where do I sign up? How do we do this?

He wrote down an address. He'd see me Sunday morning at 8am. I should be on time.

I was early.

He began by teaching the Tai Qi Dao Yin qigong form without any preliminary explanation. It was best to feel first and know later, he said. I didn't feel anything. I was disappointed and thought I just didn't have whatever the knack was. That wasn't it, he said. I'd likely not feel much in the beginning because my body was weak. Most beginners feel qi along the surface of their skin before sensing it more deeply in their organs and structures. My qi wasn't rising to the surface of my body; it was needed in my organs, my blood, and especially my bone marrow, places deeper than most of my sensory nerves. Keep doing the movements. You will feel something. You're alive.

It took five and a half weeks of daily, sometimes twice daily, practice, before I started to feel the tingling and warm sensations that many people report when first feeling qi. It happened to coincide with a check-up at the hospital.

My blood pressure was normal, the bone was filling in nicely. I had regained a little weight and, while we were on the subject, I reported I had been sleeping better too. The scans showed no advancing activity of any of the growths anywhere in my body. All good signs.

I went straight to see Tom and told him. He was happy but not at all surprised. Keep practicing, he said.

I did, and became something of pest. Whenever I had free time I asked lots of questions. Most he answered, some he ignored, and for some he directed me to ways of finding the answers myself.

I went back to finish a university degree, seeing Tom on the occasional weekend and break. He taught, advised, and subtly influenced. Slowly I came to the conclusion that there was nothing as interesting to me than qi and how it worked.

After graduation I got a job at a financial institution but otherwise threw myself into qigong training, Chinese medical theory, and as much of the philosophy connected with it that I could find in English.

Eventually, we went to China (1992), so that I could be introduced to and learn from one of Tom's teachers. We learned what we could from people Tom was connected with, went on to Hong Kong, and, a year later, were off to Taiwan on a similar expedition.

Boston, as it turned out, offered a great deal in the way of qigong training. It had a vibrant Chinatown and many generous people willing to teach (unlike the rivalries I would hear of and, later, experience). It was like a 1920s Paris of qigong.

Training consisted of long periods of repetition punctuated by moments of breakthrough. For me, the challenge was holding focus and intent while things seemed to be staying status quo. I would repeatedly discover that, even though it seemed as though nothing significant was happening, my sensations told me qi was flowing and condensing and my experience told me that once the flow and volume reached critical mass another threshold would be crossed.

I would make this my life. I enrolled in acupuncture school.

I would discover that Tom Tam was unlike most qigong masters. He did not cling to traditions. He insisted on having reasons for all he did and did not do. His way was to question and test everything. He was open to learning what he could from whomever was willing to teach, and encouraged his students to do the same. Rather than being possessive of his knowledge and students, he encouraged all of us to share what we had learned, to question it, refine it, and seek knowledge from many sources.

It was most likely his example that engendered a sense of restlessness regarding my own knowledge and ability. There was always a vague sense that there was something more, greater, with a larger scope than what I knew. We continued to search and research. Tom continued to innovate. I was still dissatisfied.

One morning I pulled my copy of the *I Ching* from the top shelf. My training and knowledge with the *I Ching* were, at best, elementary. Still, why not try? I calmed myself and allowed the qi to flow as I held my question of how to advance to a better level of training, then threw the coins that would determine the hexagram. Opening to the appropriate page, the answer was something along the lines of "What is yours will come to you. What is not yours will never come to you. So, there's no point in worrying about it."

That was annoying.

I felt the qi increase as I read "the judgement," but it gave me no other course of action than patience—never my strong suit. I put the book back on the shelf thinking, "Five thousand years of culture and this is the best I can get..."

Three days later, my sister Cheryl (my first qigong training partner and, at the time, one of my partners in a clinic we'd opened), told me a friend of ours, Sandy Ryan, had received teacher training in a style of qigong called Pangu Shengong. Strangely, as Cheryl related the story, I felt the same wave of qi pass through my body as I had experienced in the hospital, and again when I saw the sign for Tom's office.

Sandy had taught Cheryl the day before, and Cheryl said it had been powerful. I'd heard such stories many times from people, but never from my sister, and never with the qi sensation I'd just had. Sandy was due to stop by (we all often traded acupuncture treatments) and maybe I could ask her about it.

Sandy came in and I all but pounced. What could she tell me about it? What was her experience so far? Had she taken teacher training? Would she teach me? When? How about right now?

Sandy was gracious and my sister's assessment had been right. I wanted more and Sandy invited me to a group practice run by Gary Woolf, who would later become a good friend. Gary related the story of Master Ou, the creator of the Pangu Shengong style, and informed me that Master Ou would be returning to Boston to teach in a few months if I'd like to meet him.

I practiced diligently for those few months and Master Ou certainly did not disappoint. To my surprise, as I shook hands with many of his students who had been practicing for only two years, they had more qi strength than I had, then in my twelfth year of training. Part of me wanted to sneak out the back and pretend that none of this had ever happened, but the rest of me was ready to start again.

That day he taught the foundational form, which I had learned from Sandy, called the moving form, followed by the next level of Pangu Shengong, called the Non-Moving Form, and then gave a class in healing skills: how to emit qi to help others, which remains the most efficient and effective means I know of helping people.

He came back every couple of months, offering the same classes, and I retook them each time. I noticed the strength of qi-flow increased each time I took the class. Master Ou explained that there was a transmission with each class and that to retake a class with him was one way to increase ability when combined with one's own diligent practice. Still, I had no personal connection with him.

One Sunday morning I was retaking the classes for the sixth or seventh time thinking, "I'll bet he couldn't pick me out of a police lineup. First break that we have, I'll head out."

It had been a long week leading up to the class. I was tired, discouraged, and pessimistic: three attributes that don't exactly encourage a healthy flow of qi. On the break, Vincent Chu, a local legend for his Tai Qi skills and also the acting interpreter for Master Ou when he came to Boston said, "Hey, Paul." (Vincent and I had known each other for years.) "Master Ou said he remembers you."

I was surprised and looked up to see a friendly smile on Master Ou's face. Not unusual, but once directed toward me it had the effect of clearing out my fatigue, discouragement, and pessimism all at once.

"Please tell Master Ou I apologize for the other things I was think-ing." Vincent didn't pass it on. He probably didn't have to.

We began a short conversation and, in the course of it, I asked if Master Ou would consider coming to our clinic to issue qi to some seri-ously ill people we had been treating. To my further surprise, he agreed.

After that, each time he came to Boston he made a stop at our clinic to help people who needed him. During subsequent classes, in breaks, and in the generous way he made himself available to his students by inviting them to his home (he had recently relocated to California from China), he taught more than a method of qi cultivation. He taught a way of living that offered health, vitality, peace, and a unique way of understanding the universe and its history. My relationship with him has been invaluable in every aspect of my life.

Over time, I learned that he is a true Master of Five Disciplines. To explain what this means could be an entire book by itself. Put simply, the Five Disciplines tradition means to dedicate one's self to the mastery of five (or more, in his case) art forms. Achieving more than just techni-cal skill, a true devotee will practice these arts with full presence and attention. Out of these gongs (deeply devoted practices cultivated over long periods of time) the practitioner discovers and develops his or her true nature, spirit, and learns to have that presence in every moment.

Master Ou's art forms include cooking, calligraphy, poetry, philoso-phy, and he is unrivaled in emitting qi to help people heal. One of my greatest pleasures and privileges has been to sit down to a meal he's prepared. To stand in front of one of his calligraphies can be a surreal experience. He infuses his work with qi that can be felt in one's body. His poetry coveys deep sentiments, transporting the reader through a transcendent experience. There are volumes of published testimo-nials from people he has enabled to recover from life-threatening ill-nesses. He demonstrates each of his art forms with easeful grace. To an observer, it seems effortless.

I asked what made his qigong so powerful. He said that the real power of the qigong could be found in the opening lines traditionally stated before beginning the movements. "Take kindness and benevo-lence as basis. Take frankness and friendliness to heart" (translated) represents a crystallization of a deeply meaningful, profound philos-ophy. Put simply, universal, unconditional love is the primary power the creator used to create existence. There is no greater power than this love. The more we align ourselves with this principle, both in actions (how we treat each other) and in thoughts and feelings (striving for inner calm, peace, and maintaining a tolerant, gentle, and openminded attitude towards other people and in our encounters with all circumstances) the healthier we become; our ability to help others grows, and our connection to the divine deepens, leading to a more profound sense of peace, happiness and well-being.

The qigong cultivates the energy of the experience of Love, infuses it in one's body, allowing it to permeate the heart and soul. To foster this Love, Master Ou offers a closing statement at the end of the qigong: "Speak with reason, —trying not to bring harm through our speech by harsh words, gossip, and off-handed remarks. Treat with courtesy, —greeting everyone we encounter with respect and kindness, regardless of how they treat us. Act with emotion—feeling this deep love and sincerity, and acting from that place. Accomplish results—performing kind actions and striving for that which benefits one's self and all with whom one interacts."

This is how Pangu Shengong grows in power and effectiveness over time. While the philosophy is easy to understand, it is difficult to put into practice.

I said as much to Master Ou, and he elucidated: "This is a very difficult and sometimes painful undertaking. One must restrain evil inclinations, attempting to emphasize what is benevolent. Over time, the parts of us that do not align with Love will be transformed. It represents the most fundamental struggle of good and evil, with the ultimate goal being not only the transformation of the individual but of our world."

I asked if there were one best way to transform the world; would he say it was to practice this qigong? To my surprise, he answered: "The best way to be healthy, happy, and to transform the world is to try one's very best to be kinder and more loving each day. Doing this sincerely, whether one practices Pangu Shengong or not, will improve, dramatically, one's physical, emotional, and spiritual health. Over time, one's life will improve as well, moving towards a deeper happiness and sense of peace. Pangu Shengong can make it easier. However, even if a person practiced the qigong and still refused to grow in love, it would bring much less benefit."

He said striving for harmony, within one's self, with the people encountered, and with our planet is an excellent goal of any serious qi cultivation. Harmony is a natural occurrence of Love. If one wants harmony, one must contribute Love, not with ulterior motives, nor as any means to an end, but sincerely and without defined expectation.

For him, qi cultivation is not simply something one does, it is what one becomes.

In the coming years as more ancient writings on qi cultivation became available in English, and with Master Ou offering discussions on ancient culture, it became apparent that he was teaching an essential component that had been largely ignored or given superficial treatment in the works available. He sought to resurrect those teachings and make them relevant to contemporary students.

This was a new stage in the journey.

Entering it would bring profound gifts.

PART ONE

Life as an exchange with the universe

In a very real sense, the experience of living may be seen as one vast exchange of energy. Our bodies take form at conception as single-celled zygotes and through a process that, although meticulously studied remains only partially understood, the cell replicates and differentiates trillions of times until an independent functioning body is created. At some point our souls fuse together with this body, we are birthed, and we draw in energy through our first breath and offer our uniquely imprinted energy back to the universe through a wailing cry that reaches every witness to that moment when we first come into being. Those witnesses receive the energy of our cries through their ears, register it through their nervous systems, process it in their brains, and respond within their own souls: a mother may cry, laugh, and smile, exhaling with joy and relief that her baby is responding, her birthing process is completing, her heart opening with love as her body floods with oxytocin as she envelops her child in her arms, sending the energy of love, protection, acceptance, joy, and thankfulness. The doctor or midwife receives the energy of those cries and exhales as well, feeling appreciation and satisfaction, a sense of purpose and happiness at having successfully assisted the beginning of another human being's journey. The other parent receives those cries and registers love and admiration for the mother, gratitude for her safety and that of her child, and the skill of the doctor or midwife. A profound sense of love, protective instincts, and an overwhelming desire to shape the reachable areas of their world to make it as conducive as possible to the growth, education, happiness, and well-being of this new human, now in their care, is expressed energetically through smiles, tears, subtle postures of guardianship, expressions of thanks, and displays of affection. All around them they receive support and strength from the air they breathe, the water they drink, the food they've taken in and metabolized, and the people who love them. The exchange of energy is dynamic and real. Being so commonplace, it is easily overlooked, until those especially profound and powerful moments jolt us into an awareness of their magnificence. This awareness seems to amplify our sense of presence and vitality, leaving us with a reservoir of spiritual strength and energy that we may draw upon from our stored memories.

Our lives begin and gradually we develop two very real aspects of ourselves that routinely exchange energy within us, even as that energy is exchanged with other people, beings, and our world.

One aspect of us is our physicality. To support it we breathe, eat, drink, and exercise our bodies to become strong, capable, and resilient. Another aspect is our inner world, the soul or spirit. To develop it we learn, think, and feel, explore our likes, dislikes, and talents and discover how to negotiate with the outer world using our physical selves as a medium. Our inner and outer worlds exchange energy so they may grow. Our bodies send signals to our minds that we need food and water and our minds direct our bodies to acquire what we need. Our minds recognize the need to develop skills to survive like walking, talking, and taking care of our physical needs, and our bodies respond by beginning to form words, to walk, and to meet those daily needs.

As we grow and develop, our inner and outer selves become more sophisticated and the exchange between the two develops exponentially. We may discover a love of music and direct our bodies to sing or play an instrument. A joy of athletic prowess emerges and we dedicate ourselves to sports, feats of strength, and coordination. A desire for affluence may drive us to study finance or some other lucrative profession and to work long hours. An affection for another person causes us to search our hearts for ways to deepen that connection and to perform actions that demonstrate our feelings, and we draw ever more deeply on the physical strength and stamina we've developed, the material goods we've acquired, the talents we've cultivated, and the emotional depths we've plumbed.

This is life. Living it mandates that energy flows both inwardly and outwardly. If that flow of energy is relatively balanced between what flows towards us and what flows away from us, then life will flourish. If it becomes imbalanced for too long in either direction, life will be impeded.

A great deal of mental activity may take time away from exercising the body. Physical exhaustion leaves us little strength for intellectual, emotional, and spiritual pursuits. Too much desire for material wealth could cause increased mental and emotional strain, resulting in an overuse of our physical and emotional energy. This overuse draws strength away from our internal organs and we become vulnerable to disease; it takes energy away from other aspects of our lives, such as meaningful relationships and the joy we once felt in simple pleasures like playing music, watching a sunset, or sipping tea and talking with someone we love. Too much emphasis on developing a "perfect" body could result in the overuse of tendons, muscles, and ligaments; we become injured and unable to perform many simple tasks. Obsessive devotion to another person could cause us to lose our sense of selves, our definition of who we are and what we are becoming; we become unrecognizable to ourselves and those who know us.

The ancient Chinese thinkers understood that our inner lives: mind, spirit, emotions, and intellect (yin), and our outer lives: body, activity, manifestations, and material goods (yang), must exchange energy in harmony and balance if we are to have health, vitality, and a richness of experience. They examined these energies (qi) of yin and yang, devised strategies of thought, behavior, and action (gong) to facilitate this balance, and exercises to strengthen those energies, bringing them into harmony within ourselves and with the universe. They called these exercises *qigong*.

Qi is most commonly translated as energy. Sometimes it is referred to as "bio-electricity," and some publications use the term "life force" to describe qi. Each of these descriptions contains or emphasizes one aspect of qi, but a comprehensive definition remains elusive.

The chemical action for energy for cells in the body is created through the synthesis of adenosine triphosphate (ATP). While injections of adenosine are helpful with certain heart conditions, the compound alone does not restore health when it is impaired, nor will it accelerate repair in cases of injury.

The human body conducts a mild electric current of about six millivolts. Essential for survival (the SA node in the heart uses electricity to induce a heartbeat, and nerve fibers use electricity to send vital signals for organ function and to create movement, to say nothing of cognitive function), it would be illogical to suggest that qi is only a six millivolt current. If that were the case, a small battery-operated device would be all we would need to improve health and vitality, to cure disease, and to heal injuries.

"Life Force" is undeniable as a phenomenon but still cannot be examined or quantified. Once a human being dies, the body immediately begins to decay. All the material and chemical components may be present but there is no force inside the body to catalyze the actions necessary to sustain life. A qigong practitioner emitting qi to a corpse will not reanimate it. The ancient Chinese classics make reference to "life force" (shengmingli) but see it as one of three key aspects of the human soul. Qi may enhance and preserve it, but it is not equal to it.

Some publications describe qi as a large bandwidth of frequencies. Sound therapy and radio frequencies have been shown to improve conditions, and devices have been created that seem to neutralize viruses and other harmful microbes, as well as accelerate recovery from injury. (Lynne McTaggart's pioneering book *The Field* discusses many of the fascinating experiments associated with these phenomena.) And yet there seems to be a material component to qi as well: people who have cultivated qi for long periods of time have greater physical density, often weighing more than their appearance suggests; research in China has reported the regeneration of organs (especially kidneys and livers) that had been all but destroyed through disease; and anecdotal reports, too numerous to quantify, describe a "reversal" of the aging process: wrinkled appearances becoming smooth, muscle atrophy reversing, and spines becoming straighter.

For the purposes of this book, qi may be said to be a force of a large bandwidth of frequencies and tiny material particles that exist and flow through the universe, nature, and our physical bodies.

Gong does not have a precise English equivalent. Often it translates as "movement," "action," "work," and "cultivation." Inherent in the term gong is a sense of devoted presence of mind and conscious intent within an activity that takes place over a long period of time. The term

Gong Fu ("kung fu") does not mean "martial art"; this is the meaning of Wu Shu (*wu* [created with two characters meaning "to stop" and "spear or lance"] *shu* ["art"]—literally "military art"—connoting an action to put a stop to violence or the use of weapons). Gong Fu refers instead to any meaningful discipline or skill achieved through hard work, practice, and patience that helps one to discover and develop one's true nature.

The term qigong is very broad. Much like the words "food" and "exercise," it could represent many different actions that produce many varying results. We may eat a bowl of broccoli or a bowl of ice cream. Both may be wonderful experiences but will certainly produce different responses and effects. Similarly, one may train as a swimmer or a gymnast. In both cases one will become very well-conditioned, but it is unlikely that one who trained exclusively as a swimmer would be able to perform as a competitive gymnast, or vice versa.

In general terms, qigong is an art and skill to train qi, an animating current of energy that permeates our bodies and the natural world. To be more precise, it is the method by which the practitioner performs physical and mental exercises in order to calm the mind, relax the body, and then promote and conduct the smooth flow of qi. This is most often done through associating the mind, postures, and breathing in harmony with one's whole self. The effects of this practice regulate the functions of the mind and body, maintaining a dynamic equilibrium, and slowly cultivate the body's ability to "store" energy by reducing its energetic consumption through more efficient functioning, the lowering of physical, mental, and emotional resistance, and an increase of bio-energetic conductivity between cells. As the smooth flow of qi is achieved inside the body, so it also has the effect of harmonizing the practitioner with the endless oceans of energy and charged particles that surround us. From within this dynamic balancing and cultivation a person may enjoy good health and a clear and tranquil mind, and, with further training, the ability to pass on this abundance of animating current through the art of qigong therapy (Fa Gong), as well as the ability to energize the aspects of life that are more to his or her liking, and "healing" those aspects which are not. He or she may condition this current to fuse with the structure of the body in tendons, ligaments and muscle, and then condense it within joint spaces (jin), amplifying physical strength, making that person much less prone to injury, and allowing for bursts of stored power (fa jin), often used for self-defense.

Qigong has long been regarded as a mystery to some and superstition to others. Historically, qigong was treated more as a technology, one that was contained within the practitioner but could be shared with anyone. Up until about sixty years ago, much of this internal technology was kept secret, passed between family members, or given only to the most trusted students, or kept within temple walls. For many who used qigong for its martial benefits, it meant the difference between victory and defeat, to say nothing of survival. For those who used qigong for its health benefits, particularly those physicians who passed their cultivated qi to afflicted patients, often with seemingly miraculous results, qigong provided success as a physician and, in some cases, wealth and fame. There were also those who misused their skill and used their energy to harm or manipulate others, and so who could receive training depended a great deal on a master's assessment of his or her students' characters.

There are thousands of documented types of qigong and many different schools of thought. Today, they are often classified as Medical, Martial, Daoist, Buddhist, Confucian, and Transcendent. It is not at all unusual for one of these classifications to have strong elements of another, and it is highly likely that, in ancient times, these categories didn't exist in any strict sense. For example, a Daoist practitioner would very likely train in medical qigong to preserve health and to help those who were sick or injured, in martial qigong as a means of self-protection, in Confucian techniques to improve memory and facilitate learning, and in transcendent qigong to merge with the Dao, or divine flow of the universe. Additionally, there are many similarities between Daoist techniques designed to help merge with the Dao, and Buddhist techniques that help to transcend worldly desire; it is very likely that a great deal of communication occurred between these two schools, especially given that their temples were (and some still are) located in many of the same geographical regions, and both would have been influenced by Confucian ethics and the medical knowledge of the times.

The practice or technique of qigong is usually performed through one of three methods: waigong, neigong, and shengong.

Waigong, or "external practice", is perhaps the easiest to learn and perform. Similar in many ways to what people today call isometric exercise, much of it involves the working of one group of muscles against another group of muscles in a relatively static position. One key difference between waigong and standard isometric exercise is the engagement of breath and mind or intent (yi).

Typically, a practitioner would stand in a low squat, inhale deeply, and, on the exhale, flex the muscle group to be strengthened and energized. As the muscular contraction takes place, the practitioner visualizes the action he or she wishes to perform while imagining that the exhaled breath is conducted to and eventually through and beyond the working muscle groups, beyond the body, usually one to three meters away. The action is designed to condense the qi in the structure of the body, particularly the tendons and joint spaces, with the purpose of amplifying physical strength and protecting the joints from injury.

Very popular among martial artists, particularly "hard stylists" (karate, tae kwon do, etc.), these techniques facilitate unified action, the entire body moving as a single unit towards a single action, and will certainly amplify striking power and "insulate" the body with qi, protecting it from injury, if done properly. Due to the simple nature of these techniques, many practitioners will create their own forms and styles to suit their goals, but many popular and comprehensive systems already exist. Two of the most popular are White Crane Hard Qigong and *Badwan Jin* ("Eight Section Brocade").

From the perspective of Chinese medicine, however, exclusive long term practice of waigong can be detrimental. The excessive "yang" action of flexing with a strong exhale can create hypertension, migraine headaches, anxiety, insomnia, and irritability. It is said that long term practice of waigong without the balance of guiding qi to the internal organs can create an imbalance whereby the excess energy of the outer structure draws energy away from the internal organs, causing the practitioner to age prematurely. Many of these forms were designed for members of the military, usually for young men in combat, many of whom would not live to see middle age. For those lucky enough to survive, their training evolved to "softer" styles of martial and qigong practice aiming to restore organ strength and preserve health.

These practices were assigned the category neigong.

Neigong, or "internal practice", is a more sophisticated method of qigong. While waigong emphasizes energizing the structure of the body, primarily the limbs, neigong practice leads the qi deeply into the organs and bone marrow to strengthen and preserve vitality.

To do this, a practitioner will take care to keep the body as free from physical tension as possible, lowering resistance to qi-flow. Proper physical alignment ensures efficient conduction of qi and facilitates piezoelectric effects of the bones. Directing the mind towards the body's physical and energetic center, the place approximately four centimeters below the navel and two-thirds of the way in toward the center of the body (*dantien*—this concept will be explained later) condenses the qi within the internal organs. To help lead the qi in more deeply, "reverse breathing" (also called "embryonic breathing") is employed, where the abdomen is contracted on the inhale as the mind directs the qi to the center, and on the exhale the mind leads the qi out through the limbs, as if one is exhaling out of the limbs.

Medical or healing styles of qigong are generally considered forms of Neigong that guide the qi into the organs for health, recovery, and longevity. Much of what is now considered acupuncture theory is derived from the practice of Neigong, with ancient practitioners reaching such high levels of skill that the parts of the body that act as specific gates (*men*) for the exchange of qi with the natural world could be sensed and mapped. (They are now, in the West, referred to as acupuncture "points" and their pathways, "meridians.") Some truly adept practitioners developed the ability to see qi both around and inside the body. This occurred through an energizing of the area in the back of the head known as "The Jade Pillow" (roughly where the vision cortex of the brain resides) allowing them to see and record how these mixtures of universal and human qi fields would respond through illness and injury and the administration of herbs, massage, acupuncture, diet, and qi cultivation practices. These were later catalogued and are known as the Five Branches of Chinese Medicine, all originating from ancient practices of Neigong. Some of the earliest known writings in China, predating what we now know as Chinese characters, describe practices of Neigong.

Many martial arts known as "internal styles" were derived from the practice of neigong, particularly "post standing" (zhan zhuang) postures that condense the qi into the organs until it flows out to the structure and beyond the body's boundaries. Many of these ancient postures were strung together in continuous movements to create martial arts forms that both improve health and are excellent forms of self-protection. The best known are the four classical internal martial arts of Tai Qi Quan, Xinyi Quan, Ba Gua Quan, and the much rarer system, Xiao Jui Tian Wu Tao ("Little Nine Heaven Wu Tao"), with many techniques and styles evolving and combining from these systems, such as Yi Quan and Zhong Xin Dao I Liq Quan. While each of these systems have their founders, all of the founders were highly-skilled qigong masters.

Transcendent styles of qigong work to bring the qi deep within the original essence (jing) or inherited strength (from parents) of the body stored primarily within glands and bone marrow. As the qi flows into the original essence of the body, it is "washed" or purified of negative or vulnerable attributes. The Jing or essence is transformed in a process referred to as "internal alchemy". Through internal alchemy the jing and qi fuse together initiating what some might call a microcosmic "Big Bang," a creation of a new internal universe. For some, this new universe means having a body that ages very slowly, with legends claiming that some adepts lived as long as 800 years, earning them the title "Immortals." For others, it means the ability to combine and communicate with heavenly qi, enabling those adepts to exercise seemingly miraculous powers of healing, physical strength, knowledge of past and future events, nonlocal occurrences, and an understanding of Dao, "the way" or "divine plan" of the universe.

With this new understanding of themselves and the universe, styles of qi cultivation known as shengong, were created.

There are differences of opinion as to what shengong means. The term *shen* is loosely translated as "spirit." It also means divinity or supernatural power. If *gong* is to cultivate over time, and *shen* is divinity or supernatural power, then one translation of shengong is "to cultivate divine power."

Qi, while having the same fundamental characteristics as its basis, includes different properties depending on how it is cultivated. This is similar to radio waves. One may tune the same radio to receive or broadcast different signals or frequencies. A human body may receive or send different properties of qi, depending on a person's mindset, depth of cultivation, and clarity of connection to a particular "station" or bandwidth of qi. The quality of qi will vary with one's intention, the strength and ability of foundational qi to maintain a particular connection, whether or not someone's intent is in harmony with that particular flow of qi, and one's knowledge and understanding of what is contained within that flow of qi.

Many Daoist and Buddhist schools of qigong have Shengong practices. Many combine qigong states or practices with particular rituals. It is common to be initiated into the practice by a person skilled enough to pass on the necessary foundational qi acting as a conduit for the trainee. This may be likened to loading a program on to a computer. In this case, the initiate's body is the hard drive and the foundational qi is the program. Each time the student practices, he or she "runs the program."

Many have argued that certain religious practices could be called shengong. Some of the more ancient practices seem to have elements of cultivation, and certainly people in deep prayerful states have been known to reach the transcendent mindset that is common in more advanced qigong practices. In both cases there is an acknowledgment of a divine presence and force, and reports of miraculous occurrences from both schools of thought are too numerous to ignore. One difference may be in approach. With religious experiences one tends to be more passive, asking and waiting for the divine flow to manifest. In qigong practice, one is actively engaged in the routine while maintaining a mindset of connection to this divine flow. What is similar to both is the emphasis on proper behavior: kindness, love, a desire to be of service. There are also elements of continuous refinement of one's character.

Shengong is not necessarily affiliated with a formal faith such as Daoism or Buddhism. One very powerful style, called Pangu Shengong, was developed in 1990 by Master Ou, Wen Wei. Before he was able to create this system, he went through years of difficult training to refine himself as a conduit. The system is detailed in the book *Pangu Mystical Qigong*, and the story of his years of tempering and refinement is related in the three-volume set, *The Path of Life*.

What do we cultivate and how is it cultivated?

Qi

As previously mentioned, qi may be understood as a force of a large bandwidth of frequencies and tiny material particles that exist and flow through the universe, nature, and our physical bodies. If one is alive, it is present and active. It exists everywhere, permeates all things, is in the air we breathe, food we eat, water, trees, plants, minerals, animals—everywhere. To paraphrase the Daoist classic *The Secret of the Golden Flower*, no fish is ever aware of the water in which it swims. Similarly, very few of us are aware that we are surrounded, indeed, "swimming in" this animating force at every moment of our existence. This is a natural, rather than supernatural phenomenon.

According to modern science, there are four quantifiable forces in nature: gravity, strong interaction, weak interaction, and electromagnetism; they are vital components of qi. These forces are harmonized and eventually strengthened through the practice of qigong, most often using intent (yi), posture, and breath.

Gravity is defined as a natural phenomenon causing all things with mass to be drawn toward one another. These objects may be as large as a planet or as small as atoms and photons. The most common and

powerful experience we humans have is the power of our planet drawing objects to its center. Many styles of qigong, particularly those with
martial purposes, use the force of gravity to increase the density of
qi flowing through the body. Typically, this is done by holding a low
stance, putting stress on the supporting muscles to initiate a stronger
flow of qi down to the legs. As the legs strengthen, the practitioner will
reduce the resistance to the flow of qi by relaxing the body as much as
possible while still maintaining proper alignment, "settling" into the
posture(s), and directing attention (typically one to two meters, as a
beginning) below where the feet make contact with the ground or floor.
This is referred to as "rooting" the qi. Due to its drawing nature, the
force of gravity may be considered yin, and the force required to coun-
teract it by keeping us from falling, yang.

As the qi descends into the earth it combines with the qi of the earth
and these two living forces become mutually supportive over time. This
may be considered as a relationship that takes time to develop. The
deeper the relationship, the greater the development of mutual support
and communication. Practitioners often relate deeply emotional connec-
tions with the planet, an increase in respect, and a desire to preserve and
protect it. Similarly, the earth may lend assistance, increasing the dense
quality of qi-flow that protects one from injury: from a fall, a strike, or
some other form of impact that draws its power from the force of gravity. Those who have reached a profound level of this type of connection
are said to develop "iron body," a body relatively impervious to many
impact-related injuries. The Shao Lin monks are renowned for their iron
body skills and have given countless demonstrations of this capacity,
refined through serious training, such as repelling hand, fist, kick, and
weapon (including blades) strikes whilst holding these deep postures.

On a more emotional and spiritual plane, these postures teach mastery over our more primal responses of anger and fear. The pain caused
by holding these postures alerts the survival mechanism in the brain
(amygdala) and directs an impulse to relieve the pain by releasing
the stance. The more rational parts of the brain are used to override
this impulse. The more this is practiced, the greater the mastery over
our impulses that is developed. While fear and anger cause the qi to
rise quickly in the body (causing an increase in blood pressure, heart
rate, and a narrowing of vision), the deep posture directs the qi downward (eventually lowering blood pressure, heart rate, and broadening

vision). These postures are considered by many as a valuable first step in spiritual development.

Many systems that emphasize the force of gravity pay close attention to other planetary bodies that affect us: The sun, moon, planets of our solar system, and positions of constellations are often carefully considered to maximize the effects of qigong practice. For this reason, it is not uncommon for many qigong masters to be skilled astrologers.

Strong interaction, also known as "strong nuclear force" and "bonding force", is responsible for binding together the fundamental particles of matter to form larger particles. In short, it is the reason matter does not split apart due to the electromagnetic repulsive tension between positively charged protons in the nucleus of an atom. It is also one of the reasons we, as humans, have and maintain a physical body. From a Daoist understanding, it may be considered a yang energy or force of manifestation.

Chinese medical theory recognizes the different organs and systems in a body but asserts it is the qi flowing through them all that causes them to function as the cohesive entity we call a body. The term "holistic", often applied to Chinese Medicine, is understood as parts so intimately interconnected that they are explicable only by referencing the whole. As one of the Five Branches of Chinese Medicine, qigong theory applies this understanding to action. In practice, qigong movements and breathing are performed with an awareness of and application towards the entire body as a whole. Many of the movements are generated from the waist, with attention beginning in the abdominal center (dantien) and expanding through the torso, out from the limbs, and beyond the body. Similarly, when a practitioner uses breath and intent to "lead the qi," it is with the sensation that the breath fills the entire body, either through inhaling to the dantien and exhaling throughout the body, or through inhaling through all the pores to the central column of energy (called the *chong* or "Thrusting Vessel") and exhaling either through the pores or through the soles of the feet into the ground. This awareness and intent utilize the strong interaction portion of qi to enhance the harmonious exchange and flow of qi throughout the body and with the natural world. For health purposes, it strengthens the flow of qi in the organs, maintaining and enhancing health and balance. For martial purposes, it condenses the qi around vital organs and structures, creating the sensation of an inflated tire cushioning the body from impact.

Weak interaction, also known as "weak nuclear force" or "decaying force", is responsible for things coming apart or dissipating. Yin in nature, it is the reason a corpse decays, a body ages, and all matter returns to its source. It is this part of qi that induces calm, relaxation, and the ability to rest and heal.

Chinese medical theory understands this force as the body's ability to break down and release harmful substances and energies in the body and mind. Dismantling the components of a toxic substance, releasing harmful thoughts and feelings stored as energy or negative qi in the body are essential to survival and evolution. In qigong practice, this function is enhanced through a "softness" of body and mind.

Softness of body (*soong*) is achieved through releasing tension and relaxing the body's posture while still maintaining proper alignment. Softness of mind refers to a calm, tolerant and broad mindset, observing everything, but attaching to, admiring, and rejecting nothing. These two characteristics of body and mind are crucial to successful practice. For health purposes it allows the body to transform negative energy and chemistry. For martial purposes it creates the ability to sense danger, the trajectory of an intended attack, and the ability to "yield" or soften the body so it does not absorb impact.

Electromagnetism describes the physical interaction occurring between electrically charged particles. When this takes place a field of charged particles (an electrical field, magnetic field, light or combination) is generated. These fields may have either a negative charge (yin) or a positive charge (yang). This force plays a major role in determining internal properties of objects, binding electrons to atomic nuclei.

It is often through electromagnetism that people experience their initial "qi sensations." Tingling, numbness, warmth (resistance to current), and coolness (negative ions) are common descriptions among people who are new to energy cultivation. People who see auras are generally observing this subtle field. The colors represent the qualities of the current, often dictated by states of mind and how the nervous system responds, and states of physical health relative to the strength, weakness, and resistance to current.

A human body's electrical charge, generated from elements such as sodium, potassium, calcium, and magnesium is measured, on average, at 97.2 watts, roughly the power of a bright lightbulb. Our cells use this stored electricity primarily to send nerve signals throughout the body, maintaining homeostasis and making it possible for us to move, think, and feel.

Each cell in the body is a dipole, having both a positive and negative charge, similar to a battery. This means that cells and tissues hold a charge, that the charge may be either increased through cultivation or decreased through use. We increase this charge through nutrition, water intake, breathing, and movement. Muscle contraction requires electricity; breathing increases conduction, and current is increased through lower resistance. In qigong, this means using muscle contraction, breath control, and relaxation to increase the electrical flow, and mind or intent (yi) to direct that current through the nervous system into the body's cavities for storage. In terms of health, an increased charge prolongs cell life. As the charge increases, it often amplifies our usual physical abilities: the charge may affect the vision cortex in the brain, allowing us to see other spectrums; or the temporal lobe, resulting in psi abilities and transcendent states; or the sensory cortex, increasing our awareness of surroundings and the people in them; or in the muscles and tendons for greater physical strength and endurance; or the general field that surrounds us, giving us presence and influence, a "magnetism."

Harmonizing and cultivating these four natural forces requires conscious intent. States of mind have tremendous influence on qi cultivation, both in terms of quantity of qi and its quality.

Mind

For the purposes of this book, the term *mind* refers mainly to cognitive functions. The word "yi", which is classically used to describe this process within the context of qigong, has no direct correlation in English. It can mean intention, presence, meaning, opinion, desire, wish, thought, implication, and purpose—and much more.

There is an axiom that, loosely translated, states: "Attention energizes. Intention organizes." This is often understood to mean that wherever we place our attention, our energy will flow towards and, in some way, connect with that thing, action, person, concept, situation or sensation. The form that the connection takes depends a great deal on what is intended and the attitude of the person. Does he or she have positive feelings towards it? Is there a sense of anger, revulsion, etc.? Anxiety or uncertainty? The intentions will have a great deal of influence on how the qi flows back and the quality of the connection that has been established.

How to use one's yi is very often misunderstood. Often, the suggestion is to "focus," to employ an intention that is in harmony with the purpose of that qigong's style. For example: a practitioner has learned the Lin Family's Walking Qigong, designed to decongest the liver and metabolize tumors. Many practitioners will hold this intention, of decongesting the liver and ridding oneself of tumor growth, with a great deal of intensity throughout the entire practice. However, the consistent and intense focus actually serves to decrease the flow of qi.

"Focus" is only the first step in using yi. It frames how the energy that is absorbed will be utilized. As with any meaningful interaction, it ought not to begin and end with a first step. For example, if one calls out to a friend to gain his or her attention, hoping to have a conversation, once that friend answers, one would not call out to that friend again. It would disrupt and even prevent a real conversation. Similarly, when one enters into a "qigong condition" (described below), then sets an intention, as soon as there is a qualitative change in qi sensation there is no need to keep refocusing. To do this would be to have a "tightened mind." Since the brain and nervous system are key components to the smooth conduction of qi, a rigid and constricted mindset will obstruct and even prevent its flow. Once the connection is established, a practitioner reverts to a calm, peaceful and, if possible, happy mindset. This ease of being allows the qi to flow freely, its "bandwidth" to expand, and to settle into the places where it is most needed while removing those frequencies that are not beneficial.

As the practice continues, thoughts and feelings are sure to emerge. It is best to allow them to pass through without indulging one or another, returning to a calm state as soon as one realizes it has been disturbed. As a teacher (whose name escapes me) once suggested: "If thoughts keep intruding, just notice them lightly without interaction. They will feel self-conscious and leave soon enough."

Spirit

Spirit refers to those soulful qualities that are undoubtably present, active and, to some degree, express who we are, but are difficult to quantify. These may include our likes, dislikes, emotional dispositions, intelligence and reasoning ability, talents, and how we perceive objects, people and events.

Within the discipline of qigong, most agree that de, or "Virtue", is the key to successful cultivation.

As one's heart becomes more refined, both the quantity and quality of qi become greater. Regardless of the goal—whether this is good health, mystical experiences, healing skills, wisdom, connection to the natural and spiritual worlds, or martial prowess—active pursuit of de may be considered the shortest route to success within one's practice.

Master Ou, Wen Wei, creator of Pangu Shengong, sees the cultivation of virtue as the deeply personal development of five characteristics: calm, humility, diligence, tolerance and perseverance.

Calm

True calm is more than simple outward appearance. It is the ability to remain undisturbed, clear-minded, open-hearted, thoughtful and present even, and perhaps especially, when circumstances are not to our liking. In many ways, calm is the vehicle through which many other virtues flow and manifest. When we are calm, energy and information flow. When we are not, they become constricted.

Many may see the antithesis of calm as anxiety, impatience, and reactivity; an inability to contain unpleasant feelings and circumstances both internally and externally. Like many responses, they are conditioned, often through that which has been modeled for us in family, society, education, and media. Often these responses have become so firmly entrenched, so autonomic, that they may seem impossible to overcome. We may see our responses as unchangeable attributes, thinking, "That's just who I am." And yet, unconscious conditioning and reactions are not who we are. Who we are comes from the soul; the soul can be refined, and our actions and responses can change.

This may seem unlikely to take place in an inflammatory instance. It requires presence and vigilance. These are difficult to access when our reactions are the very opposite: conditioned and unconscious. And so we may create new opportunities for new conditioning. For example, during those times when we have more influence on our immediate environment, we may choose to make it more tranquil: gentler lighting, soft, low-volume music, minimal background noise, an avoidance of anxiety-promoting media, and a gravitation toward more peaceful activities. As we perform these activities, we are taking care to do them more slowly and with fuller attention. Taking time to do this develops new internal habits. These habits will gradually replace feelings of agitation with feelings of peace. The good feelings will strengthen and amplify if these methods can be used while practicing qigong.

Consistent practice of calm helps build a reservoir that can be drawn upon in daily activities. As calm grows, so does our awareness of when we are not being calm. It allows us the useful attributes of presence and vigilance in daily life.

The subconscious mind is difficult to understand. As we consciously attempt to develop healthier habits and responses, the subconscious may, in the beginning, seek to thwart our efforts. Many times this happens through the surfacing of agitating thoughts and feelings, seemingly at random, and especially during those times when we are trying our best to cultivate peace and calm. Strangely, to resist what we feel can create even more agitation. And to indulge what we feel can take us further from our goal. As was stated previously, allowing those feelings to be without any indulgence, action or resistance will help them to dissipate, encouraging the further realization that we are much more than what we feel or think.

Some of the benefits of calm are a happier disposition, clearer and more efficient thinking, increased creativity, harmonious relationships, better immunity, circulation, and sleep.

Humility

If calm can be a gateway to deeper virtue, one approach to accessing calm may be to examine some of the ways it can be obstructed. One of the greatest obstructions to calm can be found in a lack of humility. At first, this may not seem obvious. Many people who do not exhibit arrogance may still find calm elusive. What could this mean?

Calm is more easily accessed with a broad mindset. Frustration, anxiety, and a false sense of urgency are often the results of rigid ways of thinking. For example, if there is a particular task we need to complete, we each have our own way of doing it. If someone were to approach it differently, are we open to hearing another way, or are we instantly registering that other way as "wrong?" If someone has a different set of priorities than we have, are we willing to accept that? If we feel a particular way about something, and someone feels differently, with an alternate opinion, or more strongly, or with less feeling, have we made room in our understanding for something other than what we expect? Insisting that circumstances and people conform to our ideas is one way a lack of humility shows itself. We may or may not express our displeasure, but if we strictly adhere to a rigid mindset, we will suffer and it will be difficult to find calm.

Even standards for our own performance can disrupt calm. Certainly, in all that we do, we ought to try to do it to the best of our abilities. If we have truly tried our best, and the desired result has not materialized, does it make sense to indulge in an internally turbulent response? Suppose we want to learn something. We spend time, effort, energy, and sometimes money to learn and still we may discover it difficult to grasp. We may tell ourselves that we "should" be able to master it more quickly. Why "should" we? Because we are more intelligent or capable? Because less intelligent and capable persons have mastered it more quickly? Are we measuring ourselves against others and, in that process, forgetting to remain humble?

Often we can get a sense of our humility in how and when we speak. Does the desire to express our own opinions and feelings impatiently override our ability to listen and consider? There is a proverb that states we are given two ears and one tongue so that we may listen more than we speak. Showing patience and consideration while others offer their opinions shows respect. Respect is a key component to good relationships with people, great nature, and heaven.

Is there any person who can truly state that he or she has acquired all the knowledge and wisdom needed for any situation? Learning is endless and understanding continues to grow deeper. Bearing in mind that our knowledge, wisdom and ability are always insufficient, and that each person, situation and environment may have something to teach us, then being alert for an opportunity to learn is a good way to maintain humility.

Humility's seeming paradox is that it often leads to excellence and confidence.

To give what we hope to receive: love, respect, forgiveness, kindness, acceptance, patience, and warmth, is a way to inspire and foster those attributes in others, all while helping those attributes to grow within ourselves.

Diligence

Diligence may be regarded as maintaining consistently steadfast efforts toward what we have defined as important.

Nothing of value is ever acquired and maintained without effort. Effort requires commitment: of time, attention, energy, and action. Many people, once they decide on a goal, make strong efforts in the beginning, but later lose motivation. Why?

True diligence requires that we maintain effort in the face of fatigue, discomfort, mood, fluctuation, discouragement (both internally and externally), and uncertainty. The enemy of diligence is laziness. It is laziness that often prevents us from developing those attributes that will contribute to our happiness and to the happiness of others.

It is good to set goals that are realistically attainable. Any large goal may be divided into several smaller, shorter-term goals. Consider each large goal in terms of these smaller goals, and achieve these smaller goals, one at a time, until the attainment of what is wanted is realized. For example, a person suffering from poor health and low vitality may have the goal of health and vitality. He or she may decide to practice only good habits and put all efforts toward living a healthier life. That much change may be difficult to maintain. Knowing that four hours of qigong practice each day would go a long way to recovery, perhaps the first few days this becomes possible, but perhaps, over time, that person may find reasons or excuses not to continue with the same dedication. And so, beginning with an hour of practice each day, until that hour becomes an integral part of the day, may be a better beginning. Over time, he or she may add an additional thirty minutes, and so on, until four hours each day becomes sustainable. Then, better scheduling of sleep, better care in the preparation and consumption of food, and efforts toward practicing a calm and happy disposition may be introduced. In time, health and vitality result.

There has been a great deal written about good self-esteem and how to achieve it. One way of looking at self-esteem is that it is the quality of one's relationship with one's self. Like all relationships, it must be given time, attention, and respect. Being in good relationship with oneself means being someone you can depend on. If we make a promise to ourselves, and then don't fulfill that promise, how will we trust ourselves? If we don't trust ourselves, how will we feel good about ourselves? Self-esteem, as the term implies, comes from the self, rather than from outside sources such as another's praise or opinion. We will never feel truly confident, settled, and positive towards ourselves, regardless of what other people may tell us, if we are not a person we can trust, a person to whom we have shown the respect of honoring our agreements.

As we build the trust within ourselves each day, confidence, self-reliance, a sense of security and calm begin to take root. As these roots grow deeper, watered and fed through calm and humility, we are able to consider another person's opinion, even if it conflicts with our own or is critical of us, with serenity and objectivity. Differences of opinion are much less unsettling. We know we are much more than what we feel or the opinions we may hold at present. We have substance. We have earned it. The deep roots make it difficult to erode.

Tolerance

As we practice humility, we experience calm. As calm settles, we nurture its roots to grow deeper through diligence. Diligence helps us to discover who and what we truly are and, as a result, we become more patient and tolerant with others.

Along the sincere and diligent path of self-discovery, many of our own shortcomings will come to light. Humility allows us to face them without turning away, acknowledge them, and, with calm diligence, overcome them. Knowing the depths of our shortcomings and the great efforts it can take to transform those parts of ourselves, it becomes possible to recognize those same weaknesses in others. Having had them, or perhaps still having them while in the process of transforming them, we can have sympathy and understanding for those who, even though they may not know they are suffering, are suffering from the same shortcomings.

A lack of tolerance is the result of a narrow mind. Insisting that circumstances conform to our own ideas, or that people behave only in ways that please us, or that ideas match up perfectly with our own, are very rigid and narrow points of view. Naturally, a humble demeanor, both inside and out, is a key ingredient to remedy narrow-mindedness.

No one will ever be persuaded to change their points of view through force. At most, a person will only pretend to agree. Relaxing our posture, remaining open, patient, and showing understanding are all displays of respect. Respect is the foundation for love and friendship, for cooperation, for peace.

As humans, we all wish to be respected. Respect cannot be demanded. That will only lead to fear and distrust. Respect is earned: through giving it to others, through behaving with kind consistency, through actions that benefit the people around us. Respecting and accepting a person's level of learning, development, insight and understanding, even if they haven't reached yet to a level that is to our liking, and remaining patient and willing to help, without force or insistence, are all clear signs of tolerance.

As human beings we are all created from the same source. As such, we all have a right to be here and are all in the process of evolving. What is easy for one person to grasp, may be difficult for another. Where one has had the advantage of excellent instruction, another may have had no instruction or even poor instruction. Maintaining this broad mindset helps us to remain patient. Patience is an essential ingredient for tolerance.

The gifts that come from true tolerance are many. We have more love to give and, as a result, are able to receive more love. We feel less turbulent on the inside and have fewer conflicts on the outside. We will suffer much less and enjoy much more.

Perseverance

The virtues of calm, humility, diligence, and tolerance each feed and amplify the other. Humility permits calm, which, in turn, helps deepen humility and encourages diligence, creating a quiet confidence, fostering calm, opening the mind and heart, nurturing tolerance, which exercises humility, and so on.

Diligence in refining one's heart and soul, in cultivating one's best self over a long period of time (*gong*), is called "perseverance". If we sincerely persevere in cultivating ourselves we will have noticeable, positive results. We will feel more ease and peace, have more creativity, be able to give more love, feel more love, and perform more loving actions. This, in turn, will broaden our hearts, creating even more capacity of the heart and soul for intelligence, insight, the development of talents and skills, and the ability to relate with people.

As we persevere further, our heart and soul quality will deepen, allowing us to communicate with nature. Plants, animals, trees, mountains, rivers, etc., all carry essential spirit from the creator. If we show respect, love, calm, and humility towards nature, we may be able to develop more profound relationships with the world we inhabit.

Perseverance leads to results. Good results often act as encouragement and encouragement leads to perseverance. It is possible to see these five virtues as representing the cycle for elevating one's heart and soul.

Why would we not persevere?

There are times when we may give in to fatigue.

Physical fatigue is the result of too much output without replenishment. It is overcome with rest and healthy habits (eating well, the practice of qigong, the preservation of energy though calm, and moderate behavior).

Emotional fatigue is often the result of impatience and discouragement. Realizing that valuable, lasting accomplishment rarely comes quickly, and often comes in ways we cannot see at first, is helpful in overcoming impatience. If we can get past impatience, we are less likely to feel discouraged.

Spiritual fatigue can result from indulging our more negative aspects. Giving in to anger, hatred, laziness, intolerance, and greed (in all of its forms) can obstruct our more loving aspects. It is the loving aspects of us that grant balance, vitality, and growth. Consciously restraining the negative aspects while making every effort toward kindness, love, and generosity, even if we may not feel like it in a given moment, is a remedy for spiritual fatigue.

Cultivating the five virtues will bring peace, vitality, health, balance, and love into our lives and practice. The sooner we begin, the more progress we can make. If, at any time we find we have strayed off the path of health and happiness, all that is required is that we return to it. The results are worth the effort. Anyone who sincerely perseveres will surely see.

It is easy to perceive the effects of virtue on the physical and emotional body. One simple exercise is to ask someone to recall their most recent experience of feeling angry and ask them to describe the physical sensations that come with that recollection. Typically, people describe a tightening in the chest and stomach, a slight closing sensation in the throat, pressure in and around the head along with an increase in heart and respiratory rate. Ask that same person to shift focus to someone or something that creates feelings of love: a child, pet, significant other, favorite place, the witnessing of a kind, loving or moving moment, and then the physical sensations also change to a generally relaxed feeling, a lessening of physical and emotional tension; "opening" is a statement that often accompanies this part of the exercise.

This is one way the axiom "Attention energizes. Intention organizes," may be demonstrated. There are certainly physiological reasons for the described sensations. A rush in adrenaline will provoke the uncomfortable experiences that come with anger. Increased oxytocin in the bloodstream is likely to create a more "opening" experience. In both cases, however, these hormones were released from directing one's attention, either negatively or positively, and then the corresponding physiological responses manifested.

The states of mind and spirit play a vital role in qi cultivation. Many people cultivate harmful vibrations without ever being conscious of their actions. Indulging negative emotions increases negative qi, which has similar frequencies to disease, physical and emotional—creating diseases, growing them, and eventually cultivating them to such a degree that they take over that person, severely limiting that life and even bringing it to a premature end. Conversely, numerous studies have shown that actively pursuing more positive experiences has a strengthening effect on immunity, heart function, and circulation, regulating blood pressure, blood sugar balance, memory, learning, beneficial sleep patterns, and healthier brain function.

While some people are able to decide to be happier, calmer and, overall, more positive, this is generally not true for most and, from a qigong perspective, there is a very good reason. Many therapists and self-help teachers use the phrase "anger is a choice" or "happiness is a choice." As far as qi is concerned, this is only partially true.

If a person has spent years focused on resentment, he or she has built up a very large reservoir of qi associated with anger and resentment. It is stored, quite literally, in that person's organs, tissues, and marrow. Anything that may trigger the movement of that qi will easily create a corresponding reaction of outburst or some other negative expression. The responses of the people receiving those reactions are not likely to be positive either, resulting in the exchanging and absorbing of more disharmonious qi.

The cycle is potentially endless unless the person in question introduces, cultivates, and maintains a more health-promoting vibration. It may be very difficult for that person simply to refocus his or her mind on more positive or life-promoting subjects and actions. The "gravity" of stored resentment may be so great, circulating through that person's nervous system, activating the more primitive portions of the brain, that he or she may be unable to maintain the positive refocusing for very long, to break free of what has become an energetic orbit.

Lin, Soong, a famous qigong master, once explained to me: "You cannot use your mind to repair your mind. How can you effectively use something that is malfunctioning to repair something that is malfunctioning? Instead, begin by using your body to repair your mind. Once your mind is healthier, use your mind to enhance and elevate your qi. Then use your mind to lead that qi to a healthier body and a happier life."

Arts such as meditation, yoga and qigong recognize a conscious ability to promote health, well-being and effect positive life change, as well as the ability to bring those experiences to others. Meditation, yoga and qigong: each employs posture, breath regulation, and different forms of body control to induce the healthy universal qi to harmonize with that of one's body, transforming and releasing those vibrations that are harmful and enhancing, and storing those vibrations that are beneficial. The good news is that healthy qi is more powerful than harmful vibrations. A body is created to be healthy. Given even a minimum of material and circumstance, bodies find a way to heal cuts and injuries, expel disease, repair deterioration, and strengthen vital organs. All of this happens without, and often despite, our conscious attention and intention.

Imagine what can happen when our consciousness and actions become part of the formula.

Essentials of practice

Body

Within the discipline of qigong, the body is often used to achieve that with which the mind and spirit struggle. Where the mind and the spirit become distracted, subject to delusion, tormented by past events, or anxiously project into the future, the body has no choice but to be in the present moment, and can be used, through technique, to exchange qi with the universe.

The different formal styles and systems of qigong all have their specific methods. Most are based in a centuries-old understanding of Chinese Medicine (which acquired much of its canon through qigong masters' ability to see qi inside a body and how it interacts with the natural world).

Waigong, often called "hard" qigong, typically uses a low stance, with the spine aligned upright, the pelvis slightly tucked so that the space between the second and third lumbar vertebrae is opened, with an alternate flex, exhale, followed by relaxation and inhale. The hand, arm, and neck positions will vary according to the goal of the technique.

Flexing with an exhale produces a strong current of yang qi. The relaxation of the posture combined with an inhale allows that strong current to be absorbed more deeply into the cavities, organs and supporting structure of muscles, tendons, and bones. Usually the flexed exhale is accompanied by some form of visualization that leads the qi to the desired location and will then extend the confines of the imagery (or target of that visualization) and, therefore, the qi, out to the desired action. The inhale is designed to store and condense the qi more deeply within the body.

For example, in White Crane Hard Qigong there is a technique called "linking cannon fist." The left and right arms and fists alternate forward in a linking fashion, similar to the motion of pedaling a bicycle. As each fist comes forward it flexes on the exhale and the practitioner may visualize the power extending well beyond the reach of each fist, resulting in devastating striking ability. As the hands exchange or cycle through, the practitioner will relax the hands and inhale, imagining the current of qi being absorbed deeply into the structure of the hands, arms, torso, and lower abdomen.

In neigong the body is held much more softly. Relaxation is used to allow for a smooth, unobstructed flow of qi. If the practitioner is standing, the position is usually similar to waigong in that the knees are bent and the pelvis is tucked, but the position of the head and neck are such that the chin is slightly bowed and tucked in, the top of the head is raised slightly, and the spine is gently lengthened. This allows for the qi to travel through the "Heavenly Pillar," or spinal cord. The arms and hands are generally positioned to align specific meridians and acupuncture points with each other, creating motion through the magnetic and conductive tendencies of qi. The breathing is usually slow, steady, and rhythmic, and may be subtly adjusted to induce changes in the quality of qi (this will be discussed further in the section pertaining to breath). Generally all breath and intention flow from the lower abdomen (dantien) to the desired locations and then back to the lower abdomen. Depending on the style of qigong, some postures can be held statically and some require continuous movement, as in Tai Qi Quan.

Many, though certainly not all, shengong systems of qigong are performed from a seated posture, either lotus or half-lotus, popular among yogis. Hand positions often take the form of the various *mudras* used in yogic practices as well, and the chin, head and spine are consistent with neigong practice. Breathing, intention, and a deeply calm state are the keys to these practices, as well as a depth of knowledge pertaining to each system's foundational beliefs, practices, and goals. A relaxed body, mind, and spirit unite to create a strong field of qi in and around the practitioner.

Breathing

Many health, spiritual, and martial disciplines place a strong emphasis on breathing techniques. It is easy to understand why.

It is the oxygen provided through respiration that catalyzes most actions of homeostasis. The production of ATP (adenosine triphosphate), the chemical representation of energy in a human body, depends on aerobic activity. Blood oxygen level is a key indication of health. The lungs, through the hormone leptin, metabolize stored fat. The qi of the lungs provides much of the strength of immunity through guardian qi, the first line of defense against infection, and it also provides zhong qi, the energy that pervades the chest and supplies the thymus gland, key in the development of immune cells.

Curiously, the breath is both autonomic, in that it happens without our conscious attention, and voluntary, in that it can be altered through conscious intent. For this reason, sages have viewed the breath as a bridge between the soul (including one's individual subconscious and unconscious, and the collective consciousness and unconscious) and one's body and conscious mind. Attention on the breath and the application of yi (intention) has long been used as a means to expand one's consciousness and awareness, and with its vital role in metabolism (both chemical and energetic) has been used to increase qi-flow and storage in the body.

While there are many breathing techniques combined with intention and the various techniques of the myriad of qigong schools, they generally fall into the two categories of yin and yang, with both emphasizing breathing into the lower abdomen, called the lower dantien. As a general rule where movement is concerned, one exhales as the posture expands, and inhales as it contracts. After longer periods of practice, this rhythm may be reversed as a means of fusing yin and yang forces.

Yin style breathing is sometimes referred to as Buddhist breathing because many of the Buddhist systems of qigong employ that method.

Yang style breathing is sometimes referred to as "embryonic breathing", because it mimics the action of a fetus drawing nutrition from the umbilical cord and it is said to strengthen yuan qi, or the original qi and essence we had as newborns. It has also been referred to as Daoist breathing; many of the Daoist qigong and martial systems use it as part of their methods.

Yin style breathing is meant to be calming and restorative. It is used primarily for those styles of cultivation deigned to induce a calm, clear mind, encourage healing, slow and/or reverse the aging process, and to treat those conditions associated with stress and tension such as high blood pressure, heart disease, diabetes, immune deficiency and disorders, insomnia, headaches, and so forth.

If the breathing is used by itself without movements, a practitioner will inhale slowly and gently, expanding the lower abdomen, imagining that the breath reaches a space just below the navel (to be more precise, the distance of one and a half times the length of the middle joint of the middle finger below the navel), approximately two-thirds of the way in towards the spine from the surface of the abdomen, and then exhale, imagining the breath flows through the soles of the feet, about one meter beyond the body. If the breath is combined with movements, then after inhaling to the abdomen, the exhale is imagined to extend through the movements as well as through the soles of the feet, simultaneously.

Yang style breathing is meant to maintain and improve strength. It is used primarily for those styles of cultivation deigned to prevent illness and injury, to merge physical strength with qi, enhance martial ability, cultivate internal alchemy, and expand consciousness and the amplification of the senses (seeing other spectrums such auras, hearing other frequencies, sensing intentions, merging with the flow of qi in nature, etc.).

Just as with yin style breathing, when used singularly, without movement, a practitioner will inhale slowly and evenly, only this time drawing in the lower abdomen (dantien—the same location as mentioned above). As the breath is drawn, one imagines the qi condensing in the dantien and/or inside the bone marrow, and, on the exhale, gently pushes out the abdomen as the breath leaves the body, imagining the qi flowing through the soles of the feet, also about one meter beyond the body. If it is combined with movements or postures, the exhale is imagined to extend through the movements and posture as well as through the soles of the feet. Often with martial techniques, the exhale is longer and the abdominal push is a bit stronger (this should only be done under the guidance of a qualified instructor to avoid potential internal disruptions).

The different schools of qigong have subtle variations, many thought to be "secret," to enhance one or more of the characteristics of qi cultivation. Many styles, however, do not stress breathing at all, preferring to allow the posture, relaxation, and nature all to take their courses. The result is that often a practitioner will naturally or intuitively adjust his or her breathing to best suit the construct of the form.

The three dantiens

A great deal has been both written and said about the three cavities of the body referred to as the dantiens.

In general terms, they are cavities where qi is condensed and stored for health, strength, longevity, and the cultivation of enhanced abilities (healing oneself and others, martial skills, mystical experiences, communication with nature, and communication with the divine, to name a few.) The lower cavity is just below the navel in the abdomen, the middle cavity is in the area of the lower sternum just above the diaphragm, and the upper cavity is between the two hemispheres of the brain.

The lower dantien

Many people disagree on its specific point of access. Some say it is at the location of the acupuncture point Conception Vessel 6, named "The Great Sea of Qi," and some say it is Conception Vessel 4, named "Gate of Origin."

One way of resolving the disagreement is understanding that each point accesses a different aspect of the same cavity, each with one half of the general function. CV 6, "The Great Sea of Qi," expresses the yang aspect of the stored qi. Qi is generally considered yang (through it is, like all other things, further divided into both yin and yang) due to its animating characteristics; and original fluids like blood, hormones, and marrow, are considered primarily yin, due to their storage and expression of inherited characteristics (that come through the soul and spirit) and these are accessed through CV 4, "Gate of Origin."

To locate CV 6, measure down from the center of the umbilicus, the length of one and a half times the middle joint of the middle finger. For CV 4, measure three lengths inferior to the umbilicus. The depth of both points is approximately two-thirds of the way in from the surface of the abdomen toward the spine.

Focusing on either of the two access points will facilitate the flow of qi into the lower dantien. There are a great deal of theories discussing the functions of each point and why one might choose to use one over the other. Many of the theories contradict one another. Most theories that acknowledge both points as accessing the lower dantien suggest that CV 6 is used for strength, qi storage, the preservation of health, and martial abilities, and that CV 4 is used for transformation of one's internal environment, internal alchemy; it is further accepted that accessing one point will activate the other as well, and that the cavity's area is vast compared with the points used to initiate qi-flow, storage and condensation. While opinions vary as to the actual size of the lower dantien, the majority of scholars see it as encompassing the area between the upper edge of the pubic bone and just under the diaphragm.

The act of "sinking" the qi to this lower cavity has many positive effects.

Condensing qi in the lower abdomen clears and calms the mind by drawing excess qi away from the heart and brain. Qi that sits too high in the body tends to agitate the brain, causing random thoughts, difficulty in concentrating, obsessive tendencies, and an amplifying of the more primal brain responses such as fear and anger. It may also disrupt the heart's function, causing it to beat too quickly and the qi to "stagnate," that is, a sort of qi "traffic jam" where what should flow evenly is either moving too slowly or just barely, resulting in a back-up of qi that could, over time, cause the type of inflammation often associated with heart disease. One way the body seeks to discharge the stagnation is by sending the qi farther up in the body towards the brain, but this often causes even more agitation.

Much of the cause of qi sitting up too high in the body is the result of stress. Restoring the flow of qi in the proper downward direction is considered a remedy to stress.

As the qi flows down toward the lower abdomen, it will pass through the digestive organs, strengthening them, and removing stagnant or harmful frequencies. The digestive organs are lined with neural cells called the enteric nervous system. The intestines are often called "the second brain," due to the link of their neural cells with the autonomic nervous system and their ability to operate independently. The enteric nervous system is where key brain chemistry is produced, including ninety percent of serotonin (key in the balancing of depression and anxiety) and fifty percent of dopamine (which plays a major role in motivational behavior, and the signaling of other nerve cells). The ancient Daoists believed that this area held emotional memory, that by moving the qi through it, removing the energetic charge of emotional memories, the qi is purified through the physical and energetic functions of the small intestine's sorting the pure from the impure, the large intestine's removal of waste, thus calming the mind, cleansing memory, ensuring one is no longer enslaved by the past. This is one reason the ancient Daoists referred to the lower dantien as "The Cauldron."

These same ancient Daoists believed the very first cell of a human, a zygote as it is called today, resides in the lower abdomen (most likely due to the lower dantien being just below the umbilicus), and that the cell acts as the template for all of the other trillions of cells in the human body. Bringing more qi to the template, it was believed, created a more powerful human being.

When one practices qigong in a standing position, it is recommended that the pelvis tilt or slide forward slightly.

Rather than flexing the abdominal muscles to tilt the pelvis, the classical interpretation of this position is to allow the coccyx, or tailbone, to "hang," so that the bottommost tip of the bone points toward the ground, and the pelvic floor is parallel with the ground, positioning Governing Vessel 1 at the tip of the coccyx, "Long Strength," a powerful yang building gate, and Conception Vessel 1 at the center of the pelvic floor, "Meeting of Yin," so that both points are open, activated, and in communication with each other by angling GV 1 toward CV 1.

This action also opens the vertebral space between the second and third lumbar vertebrae, designated as the Governing Vessel 4 acupuncture point, Ming Men. Opening this space allows the qi to descend more easily, causing the qi to pass through the kidneys. It is said that the left kidney, the more yang of the two, passes its qi to Conception Vessel 6, "The Great Sea of Qi," with its qi being considered a more yang substance, and the right kidney, the more yin of the two kidneys, passes its qi to Conception Vessel 4, "Point of Origin," a point used to amplify jing, or inherited essence, which is considered to be a more yin substance.

While this point's name is often translated as "Gate of Life," a more literal translation is "The Gate of Destiny."

Kidney qi is associated with a person's will. If the qi has descended to the lower dantien, passing through and purifying the cells in the enteric nervous system, calming the mind, regulating organic function, and freeing that person from memories past, activating the strength of "The Great Sea of Qi" and initiating the transformative process of "Point of Origin," and strengthening the will through the kidneys, then, the ancient Daoists suggested, he or she is likely to fulfill his or her destiny most fully; one *lives* a life rather than having a life.

In qigong theory, this lower cavity is considered the most important of the three. Many systems do not bother to address the other two since, by filling the lower cavity, the qi naturally strengthens and fills the upper two.

If one were to cultivate one of the upper two cavities before the lower, imbalance is likely to result. This may be likened to building a structure. If the foundation or lower portion is not solid, the structure will likely lean or collapse.

If a great deal of qi is directed to the upper two cavities while the lower cavity remains deficient, a condition known as "running fire" could result, similar to today's understanding of psychosis, where the qi reverses its normal course of flow. This is, however, an extremely rare occurrence and unlikely to happen accidentally. It is usually caused when a practitioner attempts techniques for which he or she is not yet ready, most commonly in the realms of martial or mystical training.

In general, bodies will seek to balance the flow of qi, moving it from an area of high concentration to an area of lower concentration. The calmer the practitioner, the easier it is for the body to find this balance.

The middle dantien

Qi in the middle dantien depends heavily on virtue. The deeper one's virtue, the greater the quantity and higher the quality of qi that fills this middle cavity. Its strength includes strong immunity, adaptability, empathy, wisdom, and physical and emotional stamina.

The middle dantien is located between the clavicle and the diaphragm. This cavity is the primary residence of zhong qi and zheng qi.

Zhong qi is the energy that pervades and maintains the functions of the organs in the chest. Zheng qi acts as a protection against invasion, a type of counterbalance or transforming power, either against disease or an uncomfortable or unfortunate circumstance, to keep what has entered the body from affecting the functioning of the organs.

The Yellow Emperor's Classic of Internal Medicine considers the heart as sovereign of the body. It is the seat of consciousness, receiving input from the divine (shen) as a means to fulfill one's destiny in an upright and morally sound manner. With rich and balanced zhong qi, the sovereign makes wise decisions and makes the divine will known to all other officials (organs) in the kingdom (body) through the blood ("The Residence of the Spirit"), maintaining order through good health, happiness, and harmony with the Dao (the "Way," heaven's will or divine plan).

To be most effective, the heart requires tranquility. Naturally, not everyone should meet with the sovereign. An issue around trash removal isn't the purview of one whose task it is to oversee the whole kingdom. There is another official in charge of that: the large intestine.

For this reason, the heart has a protector, well-charged with zheng qi, called the pericardium, the sac that surrounds the heart, acting as gate-keeper and guard.

The pericardium determines the level to which information reaches our consciousness (heart). Angry remarks from an irate commuter who shouts and obscenely gestures in traffic ought not to reach the innermost recesses of the heart. The pericardium should deflect this energy, keeping the heart undisturbed. If a loved one has a concern that requires listening and understanding, the pericardium should conduct that energy into the intimate space of the heart's inner chambers to be considered with care, wisdom, and compassion.

A kinder, more loving heart strengthens zheng qi, permitting one to transform physical and emotional invasions and pathology, and to easily adapt to changing circumstances both internally and externally. It is referred to as an "invincible heart."

Strength and honor are required to achieve one's destiny appropriately. To do this, the lungs contain po, sometimes considered the more primal part of our nature, for physical strength, and righteous qi, the exchanging of what is good, useful and life promoting (inhalation) with what must be discarded (exhalation), through respiration.

The combination of qi from the heart, pericardium and lungs supplies power and ability to the thymus gland, located in the upper portion of the upper dantien. The thymus gland, rich with inherited essence (jing), develops immune cells that neutralize pathogenic invasion such as bacteria or viruses. It is considered part of the physical function of zheng qi and one of the body's largest consumers of zhong qi.

The upper dantien

The upper dantien is the brain, or, more specifically, the space between the left and right hemispheres of the brain. To fill and activate this cavity in a healthy and balanced way requires a great deal of very high quality qi.

Comparatively speaking, the brain consumes a tremendous amount of energy. In qigong theory, the brain is the only organ that does not store energy; rather, it draws from all other organs for its myriad functions, most especially from the heart.

Considering the brain from only a physiological perspective, it is easy to see why the brain consumes so much. Only two percent of the body's entire mass, the brain requires twenty percent of the body's blood supply. A typical brain cell requires twelve times more oxygen than other cells in the body and twice the amount of adenosine triphosphate (ATP). These figures represent a brain that is not yet actively engaged in the daily activities of planning, solving, imagining, responding, and creating. This means that at the absolute least the brain will consume twelve times more oxygen, twice the energy, and will require ten times the blood.

From a qigong perspective, the requirements of the brain are even higher.

While many may consider qi conduction solely in terms of meridians, the nervous system (fundamentally an extension of the brain throughout the body) conducts much more qi and with greater efficiency. That the meridians are given so much attention comes from the application of acupuncture to move and balance qi. Points on a meridian can be needled. Nerves cannot, and so it makes logical sense that qi-flow through meridians would be studied and recorded more extensively.

The importance of the brain and the alignment and positioning of the spine are well understood amongst qigong practitioners, however, who refer to the spinal column as "The Heavenly Pillar."

It was not until Hua Tuo, the legendary physician and qigong master of the Late Eastern Han Dynasty (creator of one of the earliest popular systems of qigong called "The Five Animal Frolics") that the autonomic nervous system was employed through acupuncture as a means to treat disease, due to his discovery, mapping, and detailing of points between the spinous processes alongside the spine. It was said that Hua Tuo's upper dantien was filled with such quantity and quality of qi that he was able to "see" inside a body, recognize disease and its stages, see where and how the qi-flow was obstructed, and was then able to communicate with nature in consultation for the most beneficial treatments.

Since nerves are so highly conductive, qi will not accumulate in the brain or nervous system, but will circulate from and to the various organs as needed. The body uses the heart, through the medium of the blood, to supply much of the qi needed in the brain, and the blood will draw its strength from the organs. The organs draw their enhanced power first from the lower dantien for quantity of qi, and then the middle dantien for the quality of qi. This is one way in which the phrase, "sink the qi to raise the spirit," common to many internal cultivators, may be understood.

When the qi reaches a high volume the brain is able to use it to enhance its functions. Normal senses such as seeing or hearing may be amplified. This accounts for many of the mystical and seemingly miraculous accounts of advanced qigong practitioners. In Hua Tuo's case, he could see spectrums that other people could not, communicate with life forms that do not possess verbal skills, yet nevertheless are aware (according to Daoist lore, through the simple fact that they were all divinely created and, as such, contain an aspect of the divine, as we all do), such as plants, minerals, animals, sun, moon, stars, etc., and was able to understand the soul or spirit of another human being to know what was required to save a life, bring that life into balance, or to enhance that life's evolution.

While anyone may develop sufficient quantity of qi to enhance brain function, the depth and breadth of those abilities depend heavily on the quality of qi residing in the heart. If the qi of the heart is enriched with the qualities of virtue, of love, kindness, compassion, devotion to the well-being of others and harmony with the natural world, then more of these abilities will manifest and with greater effect. Should one ignore virtue and focus primarily on power, some of the more primal abilities are likely to appear, such as ability to sense the presence of another person and to know that person's intention towards you. These, abilities resulting from a greater quantity of qi, rather than its quality, are generally limited to the enhancement of survival instincts and skills.

The higher the virtue, the more comprehensive the abilities. Or, to put it another way, qi that is not enhanced with virtue will mainly permeate the more primal portions of the brain, enhancing those functions, while qi that has been enhanced with virtue will expand to the many other brain centers: to the vision cortex for advanced sight, the sensory cortex for kinesthetic communication, the auditory center for hearing and knowing, and parts of the temporal lobe for transcendent experiences.

The quality of the frequency of the qi will flow towards the parts of the brain and body that most closely match its resonance, positively or negatively. This is also true for the internal organs. For example, excessive anger and frustration will adhere to the liver and create liver pathology. Conversely, a benevolent mindset and, more importantly, action, will help heal and protect the liver.

Entering the qigong state

With virtue as a base, the body as a strong conductor, the breath as a force, and the three dantiens as storage space, it is easier to enter the "qigong condition."

A qigong condition is described as a clear and present mindset, a calm and settled spirt, and a properly aligned body, all allowing for the smooth flow of qi through the body that produces corresponding qi sensations.

Many practitioners have their own methods for achieving this state, but there are a few points on which most agree:

1. Relax the body. Even if one is about to perform a "hard" qigong, a system similar to isometric exercise, a valuable first step is standing with the spine properly aligned (slight pelvic tilt, chin slightly tucked), the feet shoulder-width apart, pointing either forward or turned in slightly, shoulders relaxed down, a soft abdomen, slightly hollowed chest, fingers extended but without tension.
2. Calm, slow, steady breathing. Regardless of which style of breath one employs, it should not be labored, tight or rapid. Long, thin, slow and steady help to smooth the flow of qi and free its pathways from obstruction.
3. A calm and peaceful mind. With today's busy and stressful lifestyles, this is often a skill that many find challenging at first. Certainly, thoughts will intrude at times. This is part of the balancing process, the mind's way of cleaning itself. Allow the thoughts without giving extra attention or preference so that they may leave without hindrance. If any linger, allow that, too. Once the qi has balanced the associated feelings, the thoughts will move on to their next level of

evolution. One way of finding a relaxed mindset is simply to recall the last time it was present. The brain and nervous system have a tendency to adapt to attention. This is one reason why many practitioners find visualization to be helpful, or why "going to one's happy place" is so often suggested.

4. Take a moment to recall the intention of the practice. Each form and style is designed with different sets of purposes. It is useful to know what those are so that one may harmonize with those intentions. Some are broad, such as a healthy and balanced body and mind. Some are quite specific, such as decongesting the liver or condensing the qi in the structure to prevent or cure injury.

Typically a practitioner will have "qi sensations" once a qigong state is achieved. The sensations vary from person to person, and even according to time of day or season. However, most people will experience (even after practicing for a short time) feelings of warmth, tingling, numbness, magnetic sensations, cool, light internal pressure, or any combination of these sensations. As one's qi development progresses, so will the corresponding sensations. They may become more detailed, both dense and light, or may extend well beyond the confines of one's body.

Qigong, history and our present age

Many scholars attribute qigong as a systemized body science and spiritual art form to Huang Di, commonly known as The Yellow Emperor (2696–2598 BCE). In his book, *The Yellow Emperor's Classic of Internal Medicine* (*Huang Di Neijing*), early methods of dao yin exercise (literally, "guiding and pulling" exercise) and breathing techniques are referenced as ways to preserve health and promote longevity.

While it certainly is true that the traditional medicine of China, today understood as The Five Branches (acupuncture, massage, herbs, diet, and qigong), was given a great deal of advancement through Huang Di's study and patronage, the origins of qigong date back at least 3,000 years earlier than the commonly accepted 4,000 years ago. Archeological evidence decorating a stone vessel of the Neolithic period depicts early qigong practitioners engaged in practice. The images show priests (most likely shamanic, what would one day be understood as Daoist) in positions with descriptions of breathing methods that are still recognizable by many of today's practitioners.

That an emperor gave so much importance to qi regulation offers a glimpse of qigong's influence in shaping China's history. For centuries, rulers and people of influence sought to harness the power of qi to strengthen their authority, as an advantage in warfare, as a means of understanding the will of heaven, a method to deepen wisdom and insight, a way to care for their people, to enhance agricultural techniques, to avert natural disaster, and as a means to a more harmonious society.

The earlier imperial model describes a ruler not as one who lives in luxury, removed from the cares and concerns of the people, whose every whim is indulged and command obeyed. Rather, the ideals of at least 4,000 years ago depict rulers and officials as a "sacrifice for the people." A ruler was considered a ruler because he holds "the Mandate of Heaven." This mandate was not considered simply as power granted to an individual to use as he desires. The ability to rule had, in many ways, to be earned: through expansive knowledge (the economics of the day, agriculture, astrology, law, philosophy, ethics, medicine, and military strategy), and the demonstration of wisdom that, with hope and perseverance, comes through the synthesis of that knowledge. A potential ruler would begin studying at a very young age.

As part of a potential ruler's curriculum, devotion to the spiritual practices of the day were considered essential to preserving the "Mandate of Heaven." It was believed that a ruler first received divine power through this mandate, passed it on to his officials, who transmitted it to local authorities, who then maintained harmony among the common people. Strong spiritual links between rulers, their officials, and the people were the keys to a peaceful and prosperous society. If one member of this vital chain was out of step morally, it opened the door for disaster.

Constant connection to divine forces meant that a ruler could perceive what would bring the most benefits to the people and how the disasters of war, famine, epidemics of disease, and civil unrest could be avoided. Certainly, rituals honoring ancestors and asking for their guidance from other realms were important, as were festivals celebrating sun and moon phases, but so was immersing oneself in the cosmic flow of divine qi referred to as Dao ("The Way, or Path"). If a ruler embodied the qi of heavenly wisdom, then compassion, knowledge, and harmony were sure to follow. To immerse himself, a ruler would maintain the outward practices of decorum, ritual, and study, and the inward practices of qi cultivation and meditation to remain balanced and to receive divine qi.

Steadfast devotion to spiritual practice, ethical standards, moral reflection and consistent attention to the well-being of the populace often meant that rulers would have uncommonly long lives, despite the demands of their roles.

Ancient Chinese history offers many examples of sage-sovereigns, particularly during the periods before the nine regions of China were united as a single kingdom (chung kuo, the "Central Kingdom"), when the present-day country consisted of many smaller domains, many not much larger than city-states.

One such ruler was King Yao, who governed roughly 2,600 years ago. Becoming king at ninety-nine years old, his reign lasted for ninety-eight years. His reign was documented in one of the earliest histories of ancient China, written during the Song Dynasty (960-1279 CE). While it has been disputed by some, even to the point of being called fantasy, *The Yellow Emperor's Classic of Internal Medicine* states that an *average* human life span should be roughly 140 years (modern western science estimates the body's potential life span at 125 years), and is capable of being extended through proper living habits and qi cultivation. (Indeed, ancient documents reference one internal alchemist reported to have lived for over 800 years.) It was said that if it was reported to the emperor that a person in his kingdom experienced poverty, he would immediately go to that person, see to his needs, and apologize to him for not ruling wisely enough to keep that situation from occurring. If someone were to commit a crime such as theft, he would also apologize, saying that, as sovereign, it was his responsibility to see to the moral education of those in his care. Civic planning was so detailed that there was a reserve storage of grain that would feed the population for nine years in the event of famine.

Two other rulers, a father and son, Kings Cheng and Kang (1043-996 BCE) reigned during the Zhou Dynasty (1100-221 BCE). For forty years during their tenure their country remained free of serious crime. There was not a single incarceration.

The ideal of a peaceful and prosperous society in which art, music, philosophy, literature, and medicine all flourished was embodied in the phrase "heaven, earth, and humanity in harmony." All education, ethics, morals, and the goals of each person's subjective efforts were expected to bear this ideal in mind. Each member of society would strive to be of benefit both to him or herself and to the rest of society. To do otherwise would create a break in the vital chain of divine qi.

Personal cultivation for health and virtue were, at one time, hugely popular and considered integral to the fabric of ancient society. Few techniques at that time were kept secret (excluding the many martial techniques, which were considered to be the classified military secrets of the day), and qi cultivation found its way into myriad arts, skills, and disciplines.

Harmony began with the individual; first to find strength in body and balance of mind, then to use that clarity and strength as a means to understand the will of heaven, to permit virtue to take root and flourish within oneself and thus to extend that vitality, harmony, and virtue to the earth in the form qi-infused, heaven-inspired, agricultural techniques in harmony with celestial rhythms, architecture that conforms with the terrestrial qi-flow, art that transmits the artist's heart and soul experiences, poetry and music designed to awaken one's spirit to the beauty of human existence and the majesty of creation, and, should danger approach and warfare become inevitable, the ability to subdue a threatening force with minimal injury and loss of life. This way of living reflected a carefully considered path to cultivating the individual and the society and a means to attempt to realize as much heaven on earth as possible. While it would be an extremely difficult task to describe the society in a comprehensive way, many of the key components are still available for study and, in many cases, practiced today, although by comparatively few people.

Education

Unlike the western education of today, which emphasizes acquiring skills in order to have secure employment leading, hopefully, to wealth and prestige, ancient Chinese education's primary focus was the cultivation of virtue first, and then the acquisition of skills that would benefit the entire society. The time spent in formal education was short, roughly beginning at age five and ending at fifteen. A student would be required to master subjects such as philosophy and ethics, sacred rites, mathematics, astronomy, astrology, agricultural and animal husbandry techniques, law, the fundamentals of medicine, literature, and music. In ten years of study a student would be expected to master knowledge beyond the reach of many of today's PhD candidates.

To do this, specific qigong forms were employed to improve the memory and reasoning functions of the brain, while an emphasis on being of service to others was believed to be the quickest way to obtain and retain knowledge, as it was believed that virtue enhanced one's ability to learn.

By the time Confucius (551-479 BCE) came to prominence much of China was in disarray. He sought to restore the integrity of government and society he thought had been lost through corruption and years of civil strife, and structured an educational system based on whole-hearted devotion to society, teaching these scholarly qigong styles to his students, presumably with some of his own modifications. As a result, he is often credited as the founder of scholarly qigong, though the use of qigong in education predates him by at least 2,000 years.

Medicine

In many ways, illness in ancient times was seen as a person being out of harmony with himself, society or nature. If that imbalance was permitted to continue it could mean serious illness or death for that individual and a spreading of disease and disorder to the society.

The spread of disease was not just considered from the biological perspective, though certainly this had to be contained and avoided, but also in behaviors and actions that were toxic to other people. Simple rudeness was seen as a pathology. A person needed to be strong and balanced internally so that he or she would not respond with anger—or even dismay—when encountering the ill-mannered actions of others. For those who committed offensive acts, care and understanding were offered before punishment.

Each person saw it as a duty to maintain health and equilibrium to avoid becoming a burden to others. Daily qigong practice was the norm. A village physician would make the rounds to each person in his care, examine that person for signs of imbalance, make the appropriate suggestions, administer treatment or prepare remedies if needed, all in an effort to maintain the health of the village as a whole. The physician was paid a stipend by all members of the village, unless one or more members of the village became ill, then that member or members would not be required to pay until health was restored.

A physician in ancient times was seen as a skilled conduit of the qi of heaven and earth and one who knew how to restore people to harmony with these two fundamental powers. Training as a physician in ancient times was a distinct calling with rigorous requirements. Often a child with potential would be recognized by a master physician and, with the consent of the child (it had to be voluntary) and the parents, the training process would begin.

Five to ten years of qigong practice, roughly six hours each day, was required to lay a firm foundation. It was said that once a student could hold his or her hands over a well and raise and lower the water level with qi then it was time to begin learning the techniques of herbal medicine, acupuncture, tui na (therapeutic massage), food as medicine, and the many techniques of emitting qi to cure disease.

One's training often began and ended with qigong. As new techniques were learned, each was understood to carry its own divinely endowed energy. If the herb ginger was needed, for example, it was more than just the ginger's substance. Rather, the essential spirit contained in all living things, its divine intelligence, was communicated (in this case, through the ginger) and assimilated and understood by the physician, then administered to the patient through both the ingestion of the substance and spirit of the physician. As the physician gained clinical experience with the "spirits" of acupuncture points, herbs, bone setting techniques and so on, that energy would infuse his or her growing qi reservoir. After years of experience and cultivation, no other techniques beyond the emitting of qi would be necessary. All the needed remedies were contained within the practitioner after being absorbed and integrated through years of practice.

Feng Shui

Once the relative strength and balance were created and maintained within the individual, they would be extended to the world without in dynamic symbiosis.

The ability to harmonize with the beneficial qi-flows from heaven and earth was understood as the means to a fully realized life. With heaven as celestial father and earth as terrestrial mother, humanity was seen as the embodiment of these two essential universal powers. Accumulation of virtue through knowledge, insight, and kindness in action were seen as a way to harmonize with the will of heaven. Respecting the cycles of nature, carefully nurturing the portion of earth one happened to inhabit and diligent care for the plants, animals, and humans to which one was entrusted was seen as a way to achieve harmony with earth.

In the same way that advanced qigong practitioners could see, sense and evaluate energy in themselves and other people, they were also able to observe its flow throughout the natural world. Being in harmony with the most beneficial flows that traversed the planet could greatly enhance personal cultivation and strengthen society. Just as in a human being, these energies could be disrupted, enhanced, redirected for specific purposes, promote certain aspects of life and diminish others. With qi observed as flowing in predictable patterns, the adepts recorded these activities hoping to teach others how to augment agricultural patterns, promote health and vitality, prosperity, peace, and, when necessary, utilize the qi of terrain in defense of the country.

All living things absorb, conduct and emit energy. Earthly qi (di qi) flows in a complex network of magnetism, water, wind, minerals, plant life, and weather patterns. (Although some would ascribe weather to the realm of heaven, it may be considered earthly because it remains within the Earth's atmosphere, similar to wei qi, the qi emanating from the skin of a human being.) Just as a human body has gates (points) where specific frequencies of qi gather and exchange, the Earth has areas of greater and lesser qi concentration: yin and yang vortices, places where life-promoting qi is greater, where life-negating qi is expelled, and places that infuse its inhabitants with specific strengths, characteristics, and affinity for understanding the natural and divine. The study of the art and science of how humans may harmonize with di qi for greater health, prosperity, wisdom, good government, and fulfillment is known as *Feng Shui.*

The literal translation of Feng Shui is "wind and water." Good air and water quality are essential to the fostering of living beings, making these terms a shorthand for the study of earthly qi. Formal scholarship of Feng Shui is assumed to begin with Guo Pu of the Jin Dynasty (276-324 CE), author of *The Book of Burying The Dead*, though its practice was well underway for at least 1,000 years previously, and probably longer. Today referred to as the "Yin School" of Feng Shui, this volume deals primarily with proper decorum, combined with choosing the most beneficial location in the burying of one's ancestors.

While focusing on the dead to enhance the living may seem like an odd enterprise, Chinese Medicine may offer a partial explanation.

The bones contain marrow, a substance considered to house jing, the strength and characteristics that are inherited. Even after a soul has left a body, traces of jing and qi remain in the bones (one explanation for the use of bones in making early acupuncture needles). Placing the bones in the earth allows the earth to absorb and use, almost like fertilizer, the unrefined aspects of jing and qi left in the bones, and to amplify those aspects that have been refined. It is thought that there is an energetic link between substances that are shared. (Even today people share meals and drinks together as a means developing and strengthening bonds.) If part of that substance evolves and is amplified through a strong qi-flow it is thought that a similar evolution will be initiated where that same substance resides in other people. (There are treatment protocols in Chinese Medicine that employ this theory, especially in treating infants. Mother and child are so bonded in the early stages of life that it is difficult to separate the qi-flow of one from the other. If the baby is colicky, for instance, a skilled acupuncturist may treat the digestive system of the mother to resolve the colic in the child.) Care for the remains of ancestors, in placing them where the positive earthly qi-flow was powerful, was considered a way to cleanse a family's karma and to strengthen the beneficial qi that flowed throughout the family.

Some comparisons have been made with certain sects of Buddhism that house the bones of those monks who have attained enlightenment within the walls of the meditation hall. Some have speculated that the ringing of a bell, a gong, and chanting all create vibrations that reach the bones to release the frequency of the energies stored within, allowing those monks to continue to "teach" even after their time on earth has been completed.

The Yang school of Feng Shui deals with the location and orientation of buildings to harmonize with earthly qi, and then with the choices and arrangements of objects inside those structures to enhance the qi's beneficial aspects. Care and attention are given to objects as they may or may not resonate in shape, color, or usage with the qi of the people who live in that home. It is said that a true master of Feng Shui must have expertise in qigong, Chinese Medicine, geology, architecture, astrology, I Ching ("The Book of Changes"), agriculture, and military science, unless, of course, that master's proficiency in qigong is so high that all the necessary information is seen and felt. He or she will use that knowledge to direct the Six Levels of Existence (aspects that influence humanity: matter, qi, image, measurement, chance, and intuition) to the best advantages of the client.

Masters in ancient times were often the first to be consulted when choosing sites for homes, temples, businesses, and military fortifications. Entire cities were planned in this way. The Forbidden City in Beijing is one surviving example of trying to use Feng Shui to ensure lasting power. It is also an excellent example of the failure that results when technique (Feng Shui skill) is emphasized over virtue. History is rife with examples of how corruption brings disorder and tragedy to a country. The writings of Feng Shui masters are filled with admonishments that the will of heaven cannot be manipulated or subverted. In Lao Zi's *Dao De Jing* we read: "Heaven's net casts wide. And though its meshes are coarse, nothing slips through."

Music and poetry

Music and poetry in ancient China were greatly influenced by qigong theory and practice.

The ancients understood that sounds produced in nature could bring about significant responses. A sound wave is a form of energy, carrying a discernible message. A gurgling stream, birds chirping, the rustling and swaying of trees from a gentle breeze, all these may contribute to feelings of ease in the one who hears them.

Just as sound can create harmony, balance and health, the opposite is also true: the warning growl of a wild animal, a tone of biting sarcasm, shouted insults, the screech of brakes followed by metal colliding with metal... all of these are sounds produced in nature or created through human intervention that can create negative effects in the listeners. (This is one way of understanding the proverb: "Misfortune begins in the mouth.") And yet sound has the ability to promote and preserve life: the soothing tone of a mother with her infant, the soft declarations of lovers, a kind word to someone in pain... all of these produce corresponding nervous and chemical reactions that encourage the body's functioning and may reverse ill-effects from past experiences. There is even research to develop sound wave devices designed to dissolve cancer cells while keeping healthy cells intact.

Music and poetry in ancient times were meant to strengthen and heal, to inspire listeners to become better versions of themselves. It is no coincidence that many religious practices up to the present day involve music (hymns, devotionals, gospel music), or that there has often been controversy when "new" styles of music inspire rebellion (jazz in the 1920s, rock and roll in the 1950s, folk and psychedelic rock in the 1960s, punk rock in the 1970s, rap in the 1980s, etc.) One of the first actions taken by those whose established power structure has been threatened is an attempt to control and suppress the arts and media. Poetry, music, and literature have inspired uprisings, created movements, and have been among the recruitment tools of every variant of political persuasion.

Specific sounds can strengthen organs and even heal disease. Qigong masters identified six primary sounds that correspond to six organs or systems and The Six Levels of Existence, as being beneficial to health and well-being. The sounds, *xu* (liver), *he* (heart), *chui* (kidneys), *si* (lungs), *hoo* (spleen) and *xi* ("triple warmer", or the endocrine system) were, and still are, produced for this purpose.

Sun, Simiao (581-682 CE) the Song Dynasty master physician wrote:

"In Spring, breathe *xu* for clear eyes allowing wood to aid your liver.

In summer, apprehend *he*, so that the heart and fire can be at peace.

In fall, inhale *si* to stabilize and accumulate metal, keeping the lungs moist.

For the kidneys, continue, breathing *chui*, observing inner water calm.

The Triple Heater requires *xi* to expel all heat and troubles.

In all four seasons take long breaths letting the spleen transform food.

Naturally, one must avoid exhaling noisily, not letting even your ears hear it.

This practice is excellent. It will help preserve your divine essence."

With this in mind, songs and poems were composed and performed. Songs were, of course, sung out loud, and poetry was meant to be recited in a form of chanting that was somewhere between singing and speaking. The inclusion of the six sounds, the balanced tonal patterns, particularly of *ngahyin* (literally, "The Elegant Language"), an ancient form of Cantonese, disciplined breathing, and the infusion of deep sentiment created experiences that went well beyond simple entertainment; they entered the realms of universal harmony, healing, and transcendence.

Art and calligraphy

Art has the ability to transmit deep sentiments. In ancient times, thoughts, feelings, dreams, beliefs, emotions, intelligence, and ability were all considered manifestations of the soul, intangible yet undeniably real. Art was seen as the expression of the heart and soul of the artist.

Just as sound creates an internal experience that can have profound effects, visual art delivers energy and information that have the capacity to awaken souls, change perspectives, inspire, even alter physiology or remedy poor Feng Shui.

The art of ancient China is filled with depictions of humanity's harmony with the natural world and was meant to draw the observer into the experience. Many painters practiced styles of qigong specifically designed to create communication with nature. In this way the spirit of a flower, for instance, could speak to the soul of the artist. The artist could infuse that communication with cultivated qi, amplifying its message, transmitting through paint and rice paper, creating a corresponding experience in the viewer, adding nature's power and presence together with the radiance of the artist's soul: heaven, earth, and humanity in harmony through visual participation.

Chinese character calligraphy was an art form linked directly with qigong practice. Traditionally a calligrapher was trained in proper posture, loosely flowing movements subtly integrating the entire body, calming the mind, filling one's whole being with the meanings of the intended characters, and breath control—all essential elements in qigong training. Qigong forms are in many ways similar to the actions of calligraphy. Professional calligraphers were known for their vitality, wisdom, and longevity. The skill exercised with a calligraphy brush is often compared to the skill of wielding the *jian*, a traditional Chinese double-edged sword, in that both brush and sword must be made part of the wielder if they are to have any effect.

Skilled calligraphers were often sought out for their ability to infuse their art with qi. As the artist exhaled, deep sentiment, natural and spiritual connection, qi strength and cultivated virtue would flow through the artist's hand, down through the brush into the ink and onto the paper. True masters were renowned for their *fu* ("fortune") charms, characters filled with qi and spirit intended to attract the energy of good fortune. While the character of "fortune" was most often used, especially when welcoming the new year, numerous other single characters and phrases depicting lofty spiritual and worldly pursuits could adorn the walls of ancient homes, palaces, and temples. Many times a piece was placed in a location corresponding with its Feng Shui, at times to augment the good energy there, or as a "cure" if the energy was somehow blocked or afflicted, or if one of the inhabitant's astrology portended difficulties in a particular aspect of life. If one's physical constitution happened to be weak or vulnerable, for example, the character for "good health" or "vitality" might be placed on either the eastern wall or the left-most wall of the main entrance, to increase the health-promoting qi of the structure.

Some works were so skillfully wrought that simply standing in front of one could induce feelings of calm, physical ease, and an expansion of perception. While extremely rare compared with times past, there are still masters who produce art of this caliber.

Philosophy and guidance

Three books that had tremendous influence on ancient China are *I Ching, Dao De Ching*, and *The Analects*. It has been argued that none of these works could have come into being without the deep cultivation of qi and virtue prevalent in ancient times.

The *I Ching* ("Book of Changes") is perhaps the best-known Chinese classic. While there are many disagreements as to its origin, one group of scholars assigns at least partial authorship to Huang Di, the same Yellow Emperor of the classic medical text, while the majority attributes the book to four holy men: Fu Hsi, King Wen, the Duke of Zhou, and Confucius, though the appearance of the eight trigrams as a shorthand for interpreting the flow of events is found on numerous historical artifacts, many of which predate the arrivals of all of these men. At the very least, these illustrious sages contributed greatly to the philosophical commentaries and arrangements found in the *I Ching* in its current form, and without profound cultivation and deep spiritual connection the original eight trigrams could not have been used as a way to understand the archetypal forces that shape human and natural experience; little meaning could have subsequently been derived from these obscure symbols.

Many legends surround Huang Di's life and achievements. History records numerous inventions and scholarship attributed to this deified emperor. What is commonly accepted is his devotion to spiritual practice as a means of capable leadership. It is said that he cloistered himself for three years in a cave on Mount Bowang with an "immortal," an internal alchemist who had mastered qi cultivation to such a degree that he seemed to have ceased aging and could perceive the character and evolutionary progress of anyone he encountered. At first, Huang Di was refused instruction, as the master sensed too many personal concerns in the sovereign that could act as barriers to his evolution. Sent away, the emperor continued his reign while examining his own character for signs of weakness. Upon his return to the cave, rather than ask for instruction as he had before, he knelt quietly on the earthen floor and waited for the monk to speak. It was then that his deeper cultivation began.

The legend of Fu Hsi states that he was the "original human," the first created being by Pangu (the ancient Chinese term for "God", or "the creator"), and from him and Nuwa (the first female) all other humans were bred. Divine in origin and nature, it was said that Fu Hsi invented Chinese characters, hunting, cooking, and instructed humans in how to domesticate animals. Historically, he is referred to as the first emperor of China.

King Wen was the founder of the Zhou Dynasty and many consider him to be the first epic hero in Chinese history. His name literally means "the cultured king." Imprisoned as a matter of caution after the murder of his father by the Shang king, he was so respected by other government officials for his character and virtue that they offered gifts to the Shang king for Wen's release. He is, in many ways, considered the ideal ruler based on his care for his subjects, his wisdom in governmental affairs, and his genius in military science. It is he who is credited with stacking the eight trigrams to form the sixty-four hexagrams of the *I Ching*.

The Duke of Zhou was the fourth son of King Wen. He is credited with elaborating on "the mandate of heaven," stating that if rulers did not accord with virtue, but promoted injustice and decadence, it would so offend heaven that heaven would remove them from authority. Considered a paragon of virtue, the duke could have easily seized power upon the death of his elder brother King Wu, but instead acted as regent for the king's young son and the ceded power without struggle once the boy came of age. Legend has it that the Duke of Zhou became so cultivated during his lifetime that, after his death, he was able to visit those in need of his counsel in their dreams. If an important event is about to happen to someone, it is said that he or she has been "dreaming of Zhou Gong." Much of the commentary on the interpretation in the *I Ching* is attributed to him.

Confucius was a philosopher, teacher, political advisor, and official of the spring and autumn periods. Perhaps best known for *The Analects*, he described himself as a "transmitter who invented nothing." His works on morality, governing, and proper behavior are still studied, debated, compared, and are highly influential to this day. Sincerity and the cultivation of knowledge in service to others are primary principles of his teachings. His commentary on the *I Ching* is often considered the most accessible.

It was said that nature is the language of the divine. To discover divine laws, one would observe and, more importantly, deeply experience the workings of nature, their relationships with each other, and how they influence and manifest in the affairs of human society. The ability to perceive and record the recurring energies of existence requires a high level of qi cultivation, sensitivity, and profound tranquility. The book was written by those who had achieved extraordinary levels of cultivation, much in the same way as the later texts of acupuncture and herbal medicine.

The *I Ching*, simply stated (perhaps overly so), consists of sixty-four hexagrams: six, stacked horizontal lines, created from combining two trigrams. There are eight primary trigrams, consisting of three lines, each line of which may be either solid (yang) or broken (yin).

The eight trigrams represent eight fundamental forces found in nature: *chien* ("Heaven"), *sun* ("Wind"), *k'an* ("Water"), *ken* ("Mountain"), *k'un* ("Earth"), *chen* ("Thunder"), *li* ("Fire"), *t'ui* ("Valley"). Since human beings contain elements of nature combined with divine intent (soul, consciousness) these eight primary forces are very much at work in humanity, usually in complex combinations. When the six lines are stacked, they may be divided into four trigrams: The upper three, the upper middle three, the lower middle three, and the bottom three. In this way the dynamic illustrations of heaven and earth, yin and yang and their interactions, are said to be represented. To discover and cultivate one's true purpose as aligned with the will of heaven and in harmony with natural law is considered to be the overarching principle of the *I Ching*. The hexagrams are said to represent sixty-four dynamic, archetypal situations that occur and recur in nature and the human experience, offering guidance in how best to navigate.

The book was used both as a means of understanding the universe and as a method to discover the will of heaven through divination practices, most often using yarrow sticks and later by tossing coins to determine the individual lines of the hexagram, although astrology and numerology were also employed in determining the guiding hexagram. One then refers to the relevant hexagram in the book to read the "judgement." (There is also a method of using one's birthdate to find the "birth hexagram" and then, through a series of complex calculations, to discover the hexagram representing a particular time or date in the past or future.)

The "judgements" are short and cryptic. While many commentaries have been written designed to elucidate their meaning, the judgements were most likely written to convey an energetic experience, a transmission of sorts. It would be assumed that the one reading the text was experienced in meditation and/or qigong and had been appropriately schooled in morality and matters related to life enhancement. A reading is less an intellectual experience and more a matter of qi transmission and intuitive understanding, a prompt towards spiritual evolution.

The influence of this text in ancient China and elsewhere is difficult to overstate. It was used in mundane matters for business, marriage arrangements, conflict resolution, and health consultations. It guided the development of Chinese medicine, martial arts, qigong practices, Feng Shui principles, and agricultural practices. It was consulted in matters of diplomacy, alliances, military campaigns, domestic government, and public works projects. There may be no aspect of Chinese culture that has not been, in some way, influenced by this mysterious book and the highly cultivated masters who compiled it.

The *Dao De Ching* ("The Book of the Way and Its Virtue") is one of the most widely translated works of world literature. Reportedly written by the great sage Lao Zi of the sixth century BCE, it consists of eighty-one chapters written in poetic form. The first thirty-seven chapters describe the workings of Dao, the will and manifestation of heaven, and chapters 38-81 address de, virtue in personal actions, relationships and government.

Similar to the *I Ching*, *Dao De Ching* is written with short, declarative sentences and often cryptic language. In this way, the text may be used as an energetic transmission, with the phrases designed to evoke an internal experience that may be amplified through the cultivation, attitudes, and actions of the reader. Many have read the volume as a linguistic representation of qi and spiritual cultivation.

Some debate the existence of Lao Zi, whose name means only "Old Master." Legend has it that he lived for 996 years, and was, for a time, a contemporary of Confucius, and lived through incarnations of twelve different names and occupations ranging from astrologer to political advisor.

The influence of the *I Ching* can be felt and read within the pages of *Dao De Ching*. Both volumes offer a description of the creation of the universe from a witnessed perspective said to be induced while in a transcendent state. Paraphrased, they state that there originally existed the One in an undifferentiated state or chaos (wu), and then the One awoke to a potential (yiu) thus creating yin and yang, then differentiating into the four directions and the four inherent existences (space, time, matter, and spirit), giving rise to the eight primary forces (represented by the eight trigrams) and, from these, the "Ten Thousand Things," which is to say, all of manifest existence, came into being.

This description is represented in many forms of qigong today that begin with stillness (wu qi) and continue (yiu) through with intentions (Tai Qi) and movements (yin and yang) designed to mirror the above stages of creation (eight primary trigrams), a way of recreating oneself ("Ten Thousand Things") through diligent practice.

The Analects is a collection of sayings and aphorisms attributed to the disciples of Confucius. At its heart, The Analects exhorts students to develop and practice virtue through ren, the positive feeling that arises within a person when he or she acts with wholehearted devotion to the welfare of others.

When asked to expound on ren, Confucius espoused the already well known Golden Rule: "One should treat others as one would like to be treated by others." His teachings emphasized self-cultivation, imitation of those considered to have high moral conduct, and the continuous attainment of excellent judgement rather than a legalistic understanding of "the rules." Virtue was meant to be discovered, rather than taught, through contemplation of high principles and reflection on one's feelings and experience when performing actions. His teachings were conveyed more through allusion and innuendo rather than argument and persuasion, emphasizing a "soft style" approach leading to gradual knowledge and understanding. Personal example was one of his strongest tools.

A devoted practitioner of qigong, Confucius would have been well aware, through his training and his experience, that the energy one emits towards others will surely take root and effect oneself. As well as the Golden Rule, the maxim "attention energizes, intention organizes" can be gleaned from The Analects. In short, one becomes what one emits, and one emits what one has cultivated.

The predominance of the teachings of these and related texts, based upon qi and spiritual cultivation, in ancient China, shaped an unusual foreign policy. While many sought to unify China's various regions and so fought amongst themselves, invasion and colonization were considered contrary to The Way, and so were rarely pursued. (There is certainly some dispute over this assertion, as parts of present-day Korea and Vietnam were considered by some Chinese rulers to be part of China and were forcibly occupied, and after China was defeated by the Mongols, forming the Yuan Dynasty, Chinese soldiers were used as part of that empire's expansion, to say nothing of several border disputes that eventually erupted into full-scale wars with Russia.)

In ancient times, naval forces were used primarily as a defense against invasion and as protection for vessels seeking trade with other countries. In general, ancient Chinese empires invaded and colonized far less than the Western powers of the same historical periods.

Military applications

There is no major school of Chinese martial arts that does not employ a deep understanding of qi cultivation and function. While some of the inner teachings have been lost, or misunderstood or weakened through poor instruction, knowledge of their relationship to Chinese medical theory makes those applications re-discoverable. Without this knowledge many of the positions and movements become empty, pointless, and even dangerous in a martial situation.

In ancient times, basic qigong theory was very common, making it possible, based on their fundamental knowledge, for some rejected students to spy on training sessions and learn skills in that way. The secrecy that surrounds many qigong and martial styles can be understood through historical context, that much of it was considered military intelligence and could mean the difference between defeat and victory.

There are so many legends surrounding the applications of qigong for military victory that it is nearly impossible to separate fact from fiction. What is known is that as early as the Han Dynasty, qigong masters were often included in battle planning. Some accounts list their responsibilities as using astrology and I Ching skills to choose a date, time, and, in some cases, commanders for battle; another part of their contribution to strategy was reading not only the topography of the battlefield but finding the flow of qi that traveled through it in an effort to harmonize troop movements with its flow. Other accounts include assessing the qi strength and fighting spirit of the opposing army, and some histories allude to teams of masters working to amplify feelings of courage and physical strength and to solidify the coordinated action of the soldiers through linking their qi fields together, while other members of the qigong team sought to invade the consciousnesses of the opposing commanders, creating doubt and confusion, then amplifying fear and attempting to dissipate the physical strength of the opposing troops.

Toward the end of the Han Dynasty, we are presented with the legendary Zughe Liang (181-234 CE) in the historical novel *Romance of the Three Kingdoms* and the recorded history of *Records of The Three Kingdoms*. In them, Zughe Liang's exploits include being able to summon fog to cover strategic movements, changing the direction of the wind to protect against an approaching fire, and stashing a cache of weapons and grain in a mountain pass several years before the battle reached that location so he and his troops were able to fight their way out of what would have been eventual slaughter.

While much of the stories that include him are likely embellished, it was well documented that Zughe Liang was highly educated both in classical studies and esoteric arts. At a young age his wisdom and skill were already well known, earning him the nickname "Crouching Dragon." As an official, his incorruptibility and care for the people attracted the attention (and often the ire) of many high officials, and prompted the local populace to erect shrines in his honor. This lead to numerous important postings before he became the most accomplished military strategist of his era, a diplomat and an advisor.

During the Southern Song Dynasty, Marshal Yeuh Fei, an adept of numerous hard style qigong systems and the Buddhist *Emei Dapeng Qigong*, instructed all of his soldiers in a qigong form that was first recorded in the eighth century Daoist text *Ten Treatises on Restoring Original Vitality*. Ba Duan Jin ("Eight Sections Brocade") was taught to his soldiers in the form of a poem describing their movements, execution, and purpose. Very easy to learn and practice, and still one of the most popular styles of qigong today, it is designed to improve the health, stamina, and martial strength of the practitioner, while, at the same time, expelling other energetic influences coming from opposing forces (including people, environment, and subconscious impulses). In addition to improving circulation and nerve conduction along the spine, it builds wei qi, the protective layer of energy that surrounds the body and assists practitioners in being able to sense their environment. Practiced in a group (as with all forms) it strengthens the healthy bonds between people.

Always outnumbered, Yeuh Fei's troops engaged in over 120 battles and were never defeated. It was said that Yeuh Fee taught his soldiers the internal martial art (which he is often, though not accurately, credited with creating) Xin Yi Chuan. "It is easier to fight a mountain than to fight the army of General Yeah Fei", became a popular expression.

Legend has it that when Yeuh Fei was young, his mother tattooed his back with four large characters: "loyally serve and protect the country." At age nineteen, Yeuh Fei entered the army, defeated many of the enemy's most feared generals, and helped resist northern tribal invasions. Sadly, as Yeuh Fei grew in fame and influence, the emperor saw him as a threat to his power and had him imprisoned and killed at age thirty-nine.

Political opposition and qigong

For those who have practiced qi cultivation for a significant period of time there are some very obvious results. Certainly one's physical health and stamina will improve. Over time, a calmer, clearer mindset develops, enhancing emotional wellbeing and reasoning ability. Many practitioners describe feelings of being more self-contained, of not being easily influenced by the moods, arguments or enticements that come their way; it is as if "you have the information without the information having you." Having a stronger, positive qi-field often enhances feelings of wellbeing in those who come into contact with it, adding, in some cases, a magnetic aspect to one's presence. For these reasons, many qigong practitioners have been viewed, at the very least, with annoyance from those seeking to control large masses of people.

The first major political movement to suppress the Confucian school of qigong and its philosophical approach to society occurred during the Qin Dynasty (221–206 BCE). Fajia ("Legalism"), often compared with Machiavellianism, set aside moral considerations and questions on how an ideal society would function and focused, instead, on strengthening the power of a central government, emphasizing a consolidation of wealth and power under a single autocrat. Li Si, Prime Minister of the Qin under Qin Shi Huang, had hundreds of scholars buried alive and their books burned, recognizing that the Confucian ideals and the examples set by those masters would invite comparison with the current rulers, leading to a weakening of their authority.

Fajia found a later proponent in Mao Zedong who hailed it as "progressive" intellectualism. During the Cultural Revolution (1966–1976 CE), among many other atrocities, classic books were banned and burned and many qigong and martial artists were imprisoned, tortured, and killed, despite regular practice of qigong for health maintenance among many members of the communist party. Mao's personal bodyguard was a master of Baijiquan, a particularly powerful internally qi-based martial art. While it was publicly asserted that qigong and the martial arts belonged to the "old society" and encouraged feudalistic practices and superstition, it was said that Mao feared being compared with cultivated rulers from ancient times, not to mention with the contemporary masters themselves.

Possessing incredible skills and many disciples, it may seem improbable that so many accomplished masters could be apprehended. Most turned themselves in, voluntarily submitting to torture and death after their families were held hostage. (Some were released after having the bones in their limbs shattered to ensure they could no longer practice or teach.) With much of their knowledge transmitted through oral tradition and demonstration, it is impossible to assess the loss of scholarship that resulted from such brutality. Many masters succeeded in escaping with their families to Hong Kong, Macau, Indonesia, Malaysia, Singapore, and Taiwan.

During the late 1980s China's communist party sought to encourage the internal arts once more, deeming them a "national treasure." Government-sponsored research and training centers flourished for a time, in an effort to regain what was lost, but also in response to the realization that with a one-child policy and an aging population, cost-effective healthcare could soon become a vital issue.

Many masters who emigrated returned to teach. Wudang Temple put out a call in 1986 to invite the Daoist masters to return and resume the training of acolytes. Hospitals devoted entire wings to qigong treatment for conditions such as cancer, Parkinson's disease, and heart disease, meticulously recording their results. State-sponsored tours encouraging foreigners to join week-long (and longer) intensive study of qigong, Tai Qi and Wu Shu became popular in regions across the country. It seemed as if China were poised to make a large contribution to the wellbeing of the world through one of the most ancient and precious jewels of its culture.

The course changed abruptly once more, however. In 1999, a highly spiritualized and politically active group of qigong practitioners of

Falun Gong staged the largest protest (about 10,000 people) since the Tiananmen Square demonstrations in 1989.

Restrictions had been placed on the group after they refused to comply with governmental requirements. As tensions increased, members were routinely harassed. Seeking redress, 10,000 people staged a sit in, followed by protests in more than thirty cities across the country. The communist party viewed the protests as a direct threat to their authority. The Chinese government's response was swift and severe. Thousands of people were detained, tortured, and killed. Qigong research facilities and training centers were abruptly closed down, despite having no affiliation with Falun Gong. Teachers of numerous styles were detained and questioned, books were banned, and the public practice of qigong was prohibited. All but a handful of state-approved qigong teachings were deemed unlawful.

Our returning need

Yin and yang are present in all objects, lives, situations, and cycles. This is also true for human society and its evolution. The last 200 or so years has witnessed some of the greatest technological advancements in recorded history. The last one hundred years has seen technology developing so rapidly that, if it were described to a person of one hundred years ago, it would have been met with, at the very least, derision. (If the automobile industry, for example, had progressed as quickly as electronics, a Cadillac would have one hundred times the fuel efficiency and cost less than a sandwich.)

As humans, we have grown our yang existences to an extraordinary degree. In the developed countries there is a staggering amount of wealth, evidenced by larger homes, luxurious and efficient modes of transportation, sanitation, instant communication, exponential computing abilities (even for an average citizen), and instant access to huge amounts of detailed information on virtually every subject. The rise in our external standard of living, however, may have come at a cost. While some may live rich material lives, many corresponding spiritual lives exist in abysmal poverty.

The average world-wide life expectancy has exceeded seventy years and yet longer does not necessarily mean better. Rates of heart disease, cancer, Parkinson's disease, and Alzheimer's are rising. Conditions that were once rare are now more commonplace. Autoimmune conditions such as lupus, multiple sclerosis, and rheumatoid arthritis are increasing, as are more obscure conditions such as chronic fatigue syndrome, Lyme's disease, food allergies, and chemical sensitivities. Seventy percent of Americans take at least one prescription drug daily.

Even our children are not exempt. Childhood cancers have increased more than forty percent in the last sixteen years. Diagnosed autism rates since 1970 have risen 812 percent, jumping fifteen percent between 2012 and 2014. Rates of anaphylaxis due to allergic reactions in children have risen 150 percent since 2010.

It is not only our bodies that suffer. Globally, more than 300 million people suffer from depression, making it the leading cause of disability world-wide. Anxiety disorders in the United States are said to be at eighteen percent of the population, with diagnoses of attention deficit disorder passing 51 million in 2015.

Add to this conditions of the spirit that are not easily quantified: a lack of meaning and purpose, the inability to distinguish what will enhance life and what will diminish it, a lack of connection and, therefore, respect for our natural world, and, perhaps most telling, feelings of disconnectedness from other people, resulting in an inability to relate with others in healthy ways.

These conditions of body, mind, and spirit could all be improved through qi cultivation.

Body

When reduced to their essential states, most health conditions can be improved through addressing three factors: immunity, metabolism, and genetics.

When one's immunity is either weak or imbalanced many ailments present themselves. At any given time, one's intestines may contain more than 200 viruses, some serious and some not. If immunity wanes, the viruses may become active. Over the long term, more serious conditions may present themselves such as cancer or as some of today's drug-resistant bacteria.

An imbalanced immune system shows itself by attacking the body, by attacking what should not be attacked, which is the case with most autoimmune conditions and chronic inflammation.

As qi-flow is increased, it permeates and strengthens the functioning of the bone marrow, where most immune cells are produced (strengthening immunity) and the thymus gland, where immune cells mature (balancing immunity). It further improves the functioning of the spleen, which governs the lymphatic system, removing excess fluid (inflammation), absorbing and transporting essential fatty acids, and producing more immune cells, including antibodies.

Proper metabolic function is essential to survival. Processing nutrition into usable components requires fifty different hormones, most of which are produced in endocrine cells in glands. As the hormones activate target cells, the complex internal workings of metabolism continue. Weak or imbalanced metabolic functions (most commonly produced by excessive stress responses) may manifest in conditions such as: type 2 diabetes, hypoglycemia, fertility issues, weight issues, immune imbalance, insomnia, chronic fatigue, high blood pressure, and heart disease, to name just a few, as well as many conditions related to brain chemistry, such as certain types of depression, anxiety, and Parkinson's disease.

Abundant qi in the body's fourteen glands optimizes their function and regulates the balance of hormones in the body. Strong qi in the liver, kidneys, and lymphatic system helps to remove excessive hormones, particularly the debris of stress hormones in the blood that can impede vital functions.

Many assume that a person's genetics are absolute. While this is partially true (it is unlikely, for example, to spontaneously change gender, eye color, or ancestry), having a genetic predisposition towards certain conditions (cancer, diabetes, heart disease, etc.) does not make it certain the condition will manifest. Some with genetic factors develop those conditions and some do not. Healthy and unhealthy lifestyles are often pointed to as determining factors. From a qi perspective, the fewer unhealthy factors one's qi must balance, the more abundant the qi may be.

One intriguing bit of science adds another possibility. When DNA strands separate, there is a tiny, photon (light) emission. Light carries frequency and frequency may be altered. Part of the huge bandwidth of human qi contains myriad frequencies. If the light that exists within the DNA strands is affected by healthy qi, and if the qi within each person were to remain healthy and strong, it could go a long way to insulating a person from genetic factors.

Mind

Having balanced brain chemistry is a significant advantage when trying to maintain a calm and clear mind. But a great deal more can be achieved through disciplined awareness of how and where one places attention than simply addressing brain chemistry through pharmaceuticals.

Similar to every other part of the body, the health of one's mind depends a great deal on how it is fed and the ways it is used. Also just like other parts of the body, states of mind may be trained to become stronger and more reflexive.

Many minds are trained without awareness. Information streams toward most of us to such a degree that many are oblivious to its influence. The social science behind sophisticated advertising depends on creating need where previously there was none (flashy material designed to show one's economic superiority: jewelry, luxury automobiles, etc.), and then developing a sense of urgency in meeting that need (if the object were obtained and displayed then we would look better, attract a particular mate, have power, influence, etc.) and then happiness is all but guaranteed (momentary satisfaction, perhaps, but certainly not happiness). Advertising, political influence, the redirecting of ambitions to serve another's desires, even simple approval and disapproval—all these manipulations depend on an unbalanced state of mind. If there were no emptiness, it could not be filled with useless data. The longer a mind is kept in an unbalanced state, the more likely it becomes that pathology (depression, anxiety, poor impulse control, etc.) will develop.

Lin, Soong once explained to me: "One cannot use the mind to fix the mind. Use the body to cultivate qi, use the qi to clear the mind and then use the mind to direct the qi." Information and states of mind are forms of energy. If this energy is beneficial to our wellbeing it will enhance states of calm and clarity. Nature's preference is that there are no vacuums; if these states of wellbeing are absent, they may be replaced with what is on hand, making us vulnerable to many forms of unhealthy manipulation. If we have cultivated and consistently cultivate healthy qi, the mind settles. Once it settles it becomes easy to recognize those things which touch upon our negative tendencies (greed, laziness, self-importance) and lead us to life-negating behavior, or to those experiences that enhance our positive tendencies (calm, love, generosity, and benevolence) and affirm the life within us.

Spirit

In most spiritual traditions it is acknowledged that, in some way, all life is connected. Some may see it as everything being created by God and therefore connected to the same source. Others see it as an ecological interdependence of all living beings. Still others recognize a spark of spirit in other living beings and people that is similar to what resides within themselves. Seen from these perspectives, healthy spirituality recognizes the connection of all life, while unhealthy spirituality seeks to separate from that connection.

Feelings of connectedness nurture kind and benevolent attitudes and actions since, with this fundamental acknowledgement, what we do to others we also do to ourselves. Feelings of separation tend to engender selfishness, desperation, and, in many cases, cruelty. What is "other" is often perceived as threatening and must be "dealt with."

The positive aspects of many faiths teach love, kindness and seek, each in their own way, to transcend those aspects (excessive ego, greed, etc.) that prevent one from becoming spiritually realized. Many religions incorporate branches that are, either knowingly or unknowingly, a form of qi cultivation through movement, breathing, or a type of transcendent imagery. Certainly some schools of Buddhism and religious Daoism incorporate qigong as part of their spiritual pursuits. While many organized religions teach an acknowledgment of all of creation as emerging from the divine, qigong practice fuels a state of calm and peace that assists adherents in achieving a numinous state. More than just an intellectual or emotional understanding of the interconnectedness of all living beings, qigong provides a kinesthetic experience of that knowledge: feeling the qi-fields of plants, trees, land, water, animals, and humans woven together in a vast, unbroken tapestry of life.

As the experience of that connection deepens, our ability to communicate with other living beings becomes greater. It goes beyond what is verbal, and is often described as a heart and soul exchange with people and the natural world. As the communication progresses, so does the exchange of qi, of energy and information, bringing vitality to the latent abilities that reside within each person, rediscovering our own humanity.

Part of the solution

In general, most actions are undertaken with the hope or belief that they will contribute to our happiness. Education, relationships, professional advancement, the acquiring of possessions, attention to appearance, exercise, and spiritual pursuits all play a role in living. If they are in balance with each other it is likely that happiness will grow steadily.

If they are not in balance, one's life may progress toward some type of pathology: illness, loneliness, intellectual and emotional stagnation, and a loss of meaning and purpose. Reconnecting with and immersing oneself in the flow of positive qi offers healing of mind, body, and spirit. As that health deepens and expands it extends outward, contributing to the collective of healthy, life-promoting qi. Life seeks to nurture itself. In this way our relationships become balanced and healthy, a reverence for the natural world emerges, and our bodies respond.

If the healthy collective were to grow, many of the problems that plague modern life could be addressed. The rise of illness would be met with health and vitality; depression and anxiety would be met with connection, love, and a desire to help one another; the damaging of the environment would be met with respect, reverence, gratitude, and a willingness to harmonize with nature. The kinesthetic experience and the recognition of all living beings existing in a subtle yet profound connectedness would help dissolve petty differences. It would be much more difficult to lead humans astray.

With a small investment of time and learning, anyone may learn to emit qi to help others recover from illness, injury, and an ailing spirit. What is more, qi is abundant, free of charge, has no side-effects, does not pollute, discriminate, or seek to harm. As part of the natural world it behaves accordingly: it nourishes and gives to all, regardless of how it is treated.

Energy and archetypes

Many see energy cultivation as primarily an Eastern purview. The formal disciplines of qigong, yoga, internal martial arts (Tai Chi, Bagua, Xin Yi, etc.) and the varied schools of meditation illustrate highly structured methodologies that have survived thousands of years, and continue to offer health, vitality, and expanded consciousness today. Is there something homologous in Western culture?

Aside from early religious practices of the Judeo-Christian faiths (some scholars asserting that energy cultivation practices found their way into early Judaism and, later, into Christianity by way of the mysticism of ancient Sumeria, cabalistic practices, Celtic and Norse pagan ritual, and ancient Greek Platonic teachings), modern psychology, through concepts presented by Carl Gustav Jung, can offer some of the experiences of qigong practice.

Both qigong and psychology find their origins in philosophy, that is, within the depths of human thought and experience. As their respective philosophic lineages evolved, disciplines were created to bring the benefits of these philosophies to the greatest number of people. In the East, many of these philosophies were expressed through movement and forms (yang) while in the West they were expressed through mind and archetypal imagery (yin).

The Jungian concept of archetypes may rudimentarily be described as referring to highly developed and recurrent elements of the human experience. These elements may be universal human experiences, such as birth, coming of age, initiation (anything from upbringing and education, to joining the military, or to the more formal rituals found in religion), and death. Also included are the common roles individuals assume in society, such as mother, father, child, sage, protector, teacher, and student; or recurring motifs in mythology, literature, and popular culture that mirror our inner and outer human struggles, such as heroism, betrayal, a quest, and the acquisition of wisdom through an ordeal. Jung suggested that these experiences follow somewhat predictable patterns. Healthy patterns lead one toward individuation, the lifelong process of realizing one's inner self. Unhealthy patterns result in psychopathy. One way to assist one who is afflicted is to discover and explore the archetype or archetypes seeking to emerge, but which may have become stunted in some way. The discovery often occurs through the analysis of dreams, artwork, storytelling or fantasy to bring those concepts into one's consciousness, explored through understanding the corresponding cultural myths in order to reenergize one's evolution. Jung felt that if we could marry the archetypes from the unconscious mind with the conscious mind (the ego) then we would have a complete and indivisible psyche. He suggested that a psyche in this evolved state could transcend space and time—a merging of yin unconsciousness with yang consciousness.

The number of archetypes is seemingly limitless. The application of archetypal therapy is both vast and effective. It has been used successfully to treat schizophrenia, neurosis, and even long-standing physical illnesses. The huge collective of archetypal experiences, in some way, may represent a massive reservoir of healing energy that can be accessed through the realization of how one's inner experience corresponds to some form of universal evolution, and that to align with it can have profound results—perhaps the psychological equivalent to harmonizing with Dao. An archetypal therapist is, in one sense, a shamanic conduit for primordial healing energies.

This concept itself may be seen as archetypal, as it contains many of the aspects of how earlier forms of qigong were developed, and is similar to one who emits qi to another in order to initiate healing. It is witnessed when anyone acts in the role of healer, using knowledge and skill to ease sickness and pain.

In Daoist thought yuan qi is the energy that permeates and connects all matter and spirit into a vast tapestry of life. In Jungian terms it is the collective unconscious (not simply bridging all minds but matter as well). In classical Chinese thought, qi is described in different ways depending on the form it takes, but it is still qi. Jung likened the human psyche to light on the electromagnetic spectrum: the center of the visible light spectrum, yellow, corresponds to what is conscious in an individual's psyche, gradually shading into red and blue, where unconsciousness (instinct, biology, and unconscious urges) resides, but all spectrums are part of the collective human experience. Both Jungian psychology and Daoist or classical Chinese thought seek to connect one to life-promoting energies, allowing them to add strength, information, and meaning, while balancing energies that could potentially manifest as pathology (to the Daoist, turbid qi; to the Jungian, the shadow).

Close connection to nature and devotion to the divine led to the ancient Chinese archetypal concepts beginning with yin and yang, then leading to the four inherent forces, and on to the eight trigrams. The trigrams, as mentioned earlier, represent eight fundamental forces found in nature and form sixty-four possible combinations. The ancients saw these sixty-four hexagrams as representing the only possible circumstances of manifest existence. If studied, they could be used to understand oneself, any situation, the past, the future, and what one could to do produce the best possible outcome from wherever one found oneself.

Realizing that these universal forces could be summoned and directed through a harmonious relationship with nature and the divine, early shamanic practices evolved into several life-enhancing disciplines. Understanding these forces led to the writing of the *I Ching*, the development of thousands of qigong styles, several martial arts systems, Feng Shui scholarship, acupuncture, herbal pharmacology, nutritional therapy, agricultural knowledge, astrology, and the eventual development of Daoism.

The summoning and utilization of these archetypal forces was further refined into *wu hsing*, "five phases" (or "elements") that represent ever-changing forces to explain natural processes often hidden from view. While cosmology, medicine, martial arts, and morality are the most common concepts explained through wu hsing, aesthetic principles, history, and social interaction are also often interpreted through this perceptive filter. In Chinese medicine perhaps one of its most intriguing applications is the concept of constitutional types.

The five phases are labeled: earth, metal, water, wood and fire, and correspond to twelve organs, six yin and six yang. With the exception of fire, which has four, each phase has two assigned organs. Earth has stomach (yang) and the spleen or pancreas (yin); metal, the large intestine (yang) and lungs (yin); water, urinary bladder (yang) and kidneys (yin); wood, gallbladder (yang) and liver (yin); fire has small intestine and "triple warmer" (or the endocrine system) (yang) the heart, and the pericardium (yin). The continuous cycles of qi flowing from one phase to the next (shen cycle) and regulating the excesses and deficiencies of those Phases (ko cycle) underlies the use of this theory in treating disease and maintaining health. It is thought, however, that each person is born with one of these phases constitutionally out of synch with the others, resulting in the formation of certain physical and emotional strengths, and weakness, offering us five archetypes of Chinese medicine.

One may easily spend a lifetime deepening one's understanding of the constitutional types. Indeed, many practitioners of Chinese medicine treat exclusively from this perspective. The following is a very brief summary; it is in no way complete:

Earth

One with an earth constitution may have a slight yellow hue to the complexion, a singing aspect in speaking, and a sympathetic disposition. When in balance, one with an earth constitution tends to be nurturing and highly intuitive in meeting the needs of others, thoughtful, prefers security, and has a strong sense of natural rhythms. Being out of balance often leads to a lack of sympathy, recklessness, a tendency to worry or ruminate, and feelings that most actions and events are somehow related to oneself.

Metal

Metal is often characterized with a slight white hue to the complexion, a weeping aspect in speaking, and a disposition that seeks what is valuable, materially, spiritually, or both. In a state of balance, one with a metal constitution will find it easy to perceive the sacred and profane, and is highly adaptable, industrious, and rational. If that balance is compromised it may lead to excessive sorrow or grief, feelings of isolation, possessiveness, and dominance.

Water

A water constitution may manifest a blue-grey hue to the complexion, a groaning aspect to speech, and a disposition that is calm, introspective, and self-sufficient. While in balance, one may be articulate, insightful, highly intuitive, and focused. At times of imbalance, fear, cynicism, and a tendency to expect the worst may guide one's thoughts and actions.

Wood

Wood is seen with a slightly green hue to the complexion, punctuated speech, and a disposition that lends itself to organization, logic, and the meeting of challenges or goals. A balanced wood constitution is often adventurous, creative, and has strong leadership qualities. Imbalance may lead one easily towards frustration or anger, indecision, nervousness, and restlessness.

Fire

Fire is seen through either a reddish or ashen hue to the complexion, an underlying laughter in speech, and a disposition that lends itself to joyful, lively interactions. A balanced fire constitution may be charismatic, empathetic, and inspiring. Should that balance wane, one may become undisciplined, withdrawn, and obsessive.

As the study of the human-embodied aspects of wu hsing deepened, the gates or acupuncture points on the corresponding meridians revealed more detailed aspects of each archetypal force, and offered an efficient means to restore internal harmony.

For example, one with a fire constitution may reach a state of exhaustion through excessive extroversion. When this happens, he or she may find it more difficult to connect emotionally with other people, even those within intimate circles. In this state even casual or superficial conversation feels like a tremendous effort. To replenish the needed emotional energy, the pericardium meridian's eighth gate or point, Lao Gong, "The Palace of Weariness", located in the center of the palm may be stimulated. (The character for *lao* signifies labor, toil, or weariness, a three-part character consisting of flames over a roof above the radical for strength. *Gong*, "palace", is a picture of a roof over a house with a window and door. Taken together the characters reinforce the need for protection of the heart or consciousness to preserve its inner strength.) The practitioner may add an outer layer of protection from the yang counterpart of the pericardium median, the triple warmer. Perhaps the fifth gate, Wai Guan, "The Outer Frontier Gate", will be used to re-enforce a boundary against outside influences that may unnecessarily draw one's attention. In this way, the fire element is restored and balanced and the rest of the body and mind resumes its dynamic, cosmic rhythm; a person may then find it easier to interact with people and will be more at ease both internally and externally, preserving emotional energy and drawing sustenance from social situations or intimacy.

Many styles of qigong seek to summon and balance these archetypal energies, creating harmony, mutual support, and expression. One of the earliest formal systems of qigong, referenced earlier, created by the legendary physician Hwa Tuo, who most likely developed it through the writings of the Daoist master Chang Tzu (369–286, BCE), is called "The Five Animal Frolics". The form is as much a shamanistic ritual as it is a qigong form. The practitioner summons the energies of five animals, tiger, deer, bear, monkey and crane through mimicking their postures, movements, and spirits (through imitating their behavior). Each of the animals is said to embody one element. The tiger, wood; the deer, water; the bear, earth; the monkey, fire; and the crane, metal.

These concepts were further developed into the martial arts styles developed at Wudang and Shao Lin Temples, where the monks summon those elemental energies and express them through martial techniques.

Xin Yi Quan, an internal martial art partially based on The Five Animal Frolics, uses five fundamental postures, corresponding to each of the elements, as a means of defeating an opponent through the ko cycle, the cycle that regulates excesses and deficiencies of energy. For example: fire may be used to melt metal; earth will contain (subdue) water; metal will inhibit wood (a tree is unable to flourish on stone; an axe takes down a tree); water will extinguish fire. When not in use as martial applications, each of the movements are a powerful qigong that maintains health and strength.

Ba Gua Quan primarily uses the interplay of the energies of the eight trigrams summoned and interpreted through movement and posture as a means to subdue an opponent or opponents. (As a martial style, there are few, if any, that can match Ba Gua's ability to deal with multiple attackers.) Like all internal martial arts systems, diligent practice also brings the benefits of health and longevity, and may even be a path for profound spiritual growth.

Tai Qi Quan, perhaps the best known qigong and internal martial style, interprets the eight trigram archetypal energies through eight postures (ward off = Heaven, roll back = Earth, press = Water, push = Fire, pull down = Wind, split = Thunder, elbow = Lake [or Valley, depending on the interpretation], shoulder = Mountain), and five phases (advance = metal, retreat = wood, left = water, right = fire, sinking = earth). Millions have practiced Tai Qi for improved health, martial skills, and as a vehicle to attain enlightenment.

The development of literally thousands of qigong styles, able to summon and utilize universal archetypal energies, speaks to the astounding levels of spiritual and intellectual achievement of their progenitors. A master would first have to perceive these flows of energy, then harmonize with them to such a degree that both their subtlety and power were understood well enough to be used to advance human evolution. From there, sufficient knowledge of physiology, human qi-flow, medical theory, the science of movement, human nature, and the resonance between human beings and their natural world would be necessary for correctly positioning the body, controlling breath, and for choosing the imagery employed to initiate the flow and accumulation of qi.

The master would further have to be able to use all of these skills while maintaining a transcendent state, held long enough for the resonance of his or her body to harmonize with the desired universal archetypal energy, forming a cohesive pattern that could be passed on to other people, similar to loading a program onto the hard drive of a computer.

(Computer science illustrates another archetypal example of delivering information and experience through knowledge, technique, and natural laws: a programmer uses binary code, 0 and 1 [yin and yang], to create complex commands and processes.)

Qigong forms and archetypes

Qigong masters of the present day still access archetypal energy, many through the fusion of accumulated culture, myth, collective human experience, movements, postures, and breathing.

Tom Tam, of Quincy, Massachusetts, created several qigong forms. One style, Da Peng Gong, uses the first chapter of the Daoist cannon's book by Chang Tzu, of the same name. In classical Chinese mythology, a *da peng* is a mystical bird said to remove misfortune, and a giant bird transformed from a giant fish is taken as the archetype from which to draw universal qi. The myth symbolizes transformation and the expansion of perception while reminding the reader that no matter how evolved one is, one's perception is still limited. The postures and movements represent the flight of this great bird (da peng) on a quest for the acquisition of strength, knowledge, and wisdom.

Perhaps one of the most powerful modern-day qigong systems comes from Master Ou, Wen Wei, the creator of Pangu Shengong, currently of San Francisco, California. The archetype that energizes the practice comes from the Chinese classical myth of Pangu, the creator of the universe (God), but with several unique twists to the original myth.

In his three volume work, *The Path of Life*, Ou, Wen Wei details his own experiences of transformation. It begins with his imprisonment during the Cultural Revolution in 1974, and his subsequent introduction to Pangu, first as a force that controls his body, then as a voice in his mind that converses with him, and finally as a mystical power that induces visions of the past, present, and future. In the beginning of the story Ou is a staunch atheist and believes his experiences are the result of a psychotic breakdown from the stress of his political persecution. Even at the end of the third volume, he does not profess himself to be a believer but, rather, only acknowledges that his experiences have profoundly broadened his worldview and have changed the course of his life.

The volumes describe events leading to the creation of the universe, and different incarnations of Earth, explaining how life was similar to and different from conditions of today. There are lengthy discussions about the origins of good and evil, the formation of the world's different religious and political systems, the eventual joining of the seemingly opposed worldviews of materialism and idealism, and the meaning of living in our present age. It puts forth an outline of a divine plan, presenting a version of the future filled with peace, abundance, and beauty.

Master Ou's purpose in recording his strange visions was to present his experiences, to discover if anyone else had received similar revelations with the hope that someone might cast some light on his implausible journey. Once the political climate of China permitted it, he self-published a thousand copies of *The Path of Life* and waited for responses.

The results were unexpected. Readers wrote to him describing many strange occurrences. When reading anything else, they remained alert, but as soon as they began reading *The Path of Life*, however, some reported falling into a deep sleep, usually lasting a short time, but would awaken refreshed and energized. Others spoke of unusual bodily sensations such as tingling, warmth, pressure, or a lessening of discomfort during and after reading. Some people had their own mystical visions.

As the letters continued to arrive, he began to receive reports of people's illnesses and injuries improving soon after they read his book. The letters raised more questions than they answered. Was it possible that simply being exposed to a unique story with an unusual message could initiate healing?

Still in touch and having frequent conversations in his mind with the mystical entity that claimed to be the creator of the universe, Pangu, Master Ou asked if *The Path of Life* was the reason for so many people's positive experiences. He was told it was. Master Ou further investigated the written and anecdotal accounts of different instances of healing, both spontaneous and gradual. China, a country with a rich traditional medical canon and spiritual history, was enjoying a much more relaxed political climate than during the Cultural Revolution. It turned out to be an excellent place for this kind of research.

His studies brought him to the topic of qigong. He wondered if it would be possible to condense the energy and information of *The Path of Life* into a qigong routine that would be easy to learn and practice, and then offer it to people as a means of helping them recover from serious health conditions. After a great deal of pondering and many hours of what he termed "negotiations" with Pangu, he created the moving form of Pangu Mystical Qigong (Pangu Shengong).

As students of this newly-created qigong began to report many positive results, some seemingly miraculous, Master Ou further considered the needs of humanity. Knowing that people are not just afflicted by physical ailments, but by emotional pain and torment as well, he created a second form of Pangu Mystical Qigong called the non-moving form. This form seeks to improve conditions of the "heart and soul," the unseen yet very real aspects of human beings, such as emotions, cognitive ability, creativity, intuition, and feelings of spiritual connection. And for those students who have an interest in helping others, Master

Ou developed a series of techniques to transmit healing energy to those in need without depleting their own supply of qi.

Thousands of people learned, continue to learn, and practice Pangu Mystical Qigong. People from many different backgrounds and cultures have shared stories of healing and transformation. The key, Master Ou explained, is the foundation of love and kindness infused in the practices and expressed in a type of mantra that is recited three times before the beginning of each routine: "Take kindness and benevolence as basis. Take frankness and friendliness to heart." The words act as a way of attuning one's nervous system to the stream of collective energy transmitted through *The Path of Life* and the universal expressions of love, healing, peace, and happiness. Simply repeating the phrase to oneself (three times) is one way to have a positive effect on one's qi.

Like many qigong masters before him, Master Ou first had to connect with this stream of energy, understand its effects, condition his body to contain and conduct this energy, and then develop a series of movements that would act as a medium of expression for such a powerful stream of qi.

Two of Master Ou's students, Vincent Chu and Anisha Desai Fraser, had extensive backgrounds in Tai Qi and yoga, respectively. Both passionate about their arts and deeply impressed with the way Pangu Shengong conducts divine energy, they asked Master Ou if it would be possible for him to infuse the routines of Tai Qi and yoga with a similar stream of qi. Master Ou worked closely with his two students to help them embody and transmit certain aspects of Pangu energy, resulting in the creation of two fusions of Pangu Qigong: with Tai Qi, called "The Returning Form of Tai Qi"; and with yoga, called "Pangu Yoga".

Using the collective of the healing archetype

The greater the number of people who employ the same sets of techniques, the more likely it is that those techniques will grow in power, creating a greater energetic collective with even more ease of access to it. Experiments in how this collective may positively affect society and the world have suggested some astounding possibilities.

The famous "Maharishi Effect" of Transcendental Meditation (TM) on crime rates, postulated and demonstrated first in 1960, is that if one percent of the population were to practice TM, then it would have a profoundly positive effect on the rest of the society. The theory was most recently demonstrated during 2007–2010, when a group of over 1725 TM practitioners (the square root of one percent of the U.S. population at that time) meditated in unison, daily. The violent crime rate in the U.S. dropped eighteen and a half percent. Before the beginning of the experiment, the assertion was predicted, released to the press, and made public that violent crime would decrease by at least sixteen percent once the critical mass of advanced practitioners took effect.

In Lynne McTaggart's book, *The Intention Experiment*, readers from over thirty countries are given an invitation to a global experiment aimed at using collective intention to improve conditions throughout the world. The goals are stated before each experiment and the results are published online at www.lynnemctaggart.com, suggesting much more than a casual correlation.

On the surface, these results may seem surprising. But healing and balance are universal experiences and are, therefore, archetypes that may be accessed. Both ancient Chinese philosophy and Jungian theory assert that we are all part of a single collective. If a significant portion of the collective focuses on a particular archetypal energy, that energy will become more active within the entire collective and the positive results will become more widespread.

In 2001, Tom Tam felt ready to put this theory to the test. Understanding that qi, the healing experience, and particular obstacles that block qi from initiating the healing experience are all archetypal—that is, common to a large part of humanity—Tom developed a technique that could be used by anyone to initiate healing. He called this technique *Tong Ren*.

Literally translated, Tong Ren means "bronze man." The bronze man replicas were first used during the Song Dynasty as full-sized representations of human beings, complete with marked indentations for 657 acupuncture points and twelve meridians, designed to instruct early medical students. The models were hollow, allowing them to be coated in wax and then filled with water. If the points were correctly needled, water would escape from the wax coated hole that represented the acupuncture point.

Qi as a means for healing, and meridians and points as a means of conducting that qi, were represented and studied on the bronze model of a man. This meant that the body of a man, the meridians, points, and the concept of qi were all understood by a significant part of the Chinese population and had, therefore, been energized and brought out of the collective unconscious and into consciousness by millions of people over thousands of years, increasing as Chinese culture and medicine were introduced to the West on a large scale in the 1970s.

Tom realized all that was needed was a method or means of focus to allow anyone to initiate a flow of qi with the intention to break through any obstructions to that flow so that, once the flow of qi was reestablished, a body would use that qi to heal injuries and reverse the disease process.

Keeping as close to the original idea of the "bronze man" as he could, so as best to access the reservoir of qi associated with that archetypal image, Tom chose to use a rubber or plastic acupuncture doll as the means of focus. In his earliest experiments he "connected" the image of the doll with that of the patient. From his years of clinical experience he knew which areas of a person's qi-flow were likely to be blocked once a disease manifested. He inserted needles into the appropriate points on the doll, and the image of the doll "reflected" the intention of clearing the blockage and initiating qi-flow back to the patient.

The first patient to be treated with Tong Ren, in the winter of 2001, had a diagnosis of lung cancer. Within a few weeks, the lung cancer was undetectable.

In order to make this technique available to as many mainstream people as possible, Tom replaced the use of needles with tapping on the points with a magnetic hammer device (considered one of the "nine needles" developed by the eastern Han Dynasty physician, Hwa Tuo), which could be legally obtained and used by anyone. He invited anyone who had an interest to come and learn. He offered all his experience, gained over twenty years, of treating patients with conditions ranging from simple colds and flu to cancer and Parkinson's Disease in an easily referenced manual. All that was needed after that, he said, was to experience the Tong Ren technique once. As soon as that happened, one was "connected" to the technique and could use it successfully.

By February of 2002, regular group-healing sessions were offered by Tom and his students. In the first three years, more than 2,200 people attended these sessions of more than sixty people each time.

The way it is offered today, participants are seated facing the group leader at the beginning of each session. The group leader will have a brief discussion with each participant to determine the nature of his or her condition and which points are to be "tapped." As the leader and assistants "tap," they seek to access the collective energy associated with the healing process. Physical contact and even close proximity to participants is not necessary. Many people have participated from other countries via an internet connection.

After the first three years more than ninety percent of regular participants, many of whom were given life-threatening diagnoses, were still alive and reported feeling very hopeful. According to many current students of Tom's, that number remains consistent to this day.

Tom believes that as more people participate and receive benefits from Tong Ren its power will grow. As more people give their attention and intention to this process, access to this healing collective will become easier, offering more benefits to more people in need.

While experience with qigong is not required to participate in Tong Ren, it could not have come into being as a technique without it. Had Tom not had years of experience in qigong, Tai Qi, and as a clinician, accesses to this collective energy would have been doubtful at best. He continues to study, practice, and teach qigong and Tai Qi to this day.

One possible direction

Qigong and the techniques that are derived from it may very well prove to be the cutting edge of medicine in the years to come. With so many conditions such as cancer, autoimmune disorders, severe allergic reactions, and Alzheimer's, to name just a few, with little or no viable treatment options, it makes sense to turn to something that has been proved through thousands of years of experience and yet still awaits the serious rigors of scientific inquiry. As human beings who are alive and, therefore, in possession of qi and the ability to acquire more of it, direct it for positive outcomes, and use it for the rediscovery of profound human potential, all that stands as a barrier is basic knowledge, which is easy enough to obtain, and a willingness to practice. The benefits have already revealed themselves. The possibilities have yet to be discovered.

PART TWO

THREE PRACTICES

There are thousands of recorded qigong practices and likely tens of thousands of practices that have never been recorded, but kept within families and transmitted orally, as has been customary for millennia. Each system exercises and develops qi in its own way. Where one may practice a particular style and have seemingly miraculous results, another may not. The reasons are many. It could be that the style in question fills the exact need of one practitioner but another practitioner's needs are quite different. A person's mindset, level of virtue, relative calm, and attention to technique may all be factors. This makes a good teacher useful, but not necessarily essential.

Before beginning any new routine, it is important to be properly evaluated by a qualified medical practitioner. Even seemingly easy movements can cause injury if a body isn't ready for them.

Each of the following exercises may stand alone as a means to develop qi, enhance health, and increase strength. For those practitioners wishing for well-rounded, in-depth qi experiences, it is recommended to build up to practicing all three exercises in order and in succession as a complete training session each day. For general health concerns and wellbeing, Tai Qi Dao Yin is recommended, for additional martial prowess, external Yi Jin Jing, for internal power and enhanced development, Cheng Bao Zhuang.

Waigong practice: external Yi Jin Jing ("Tendon Changing Practice")

A brief history

Yi Jin Jing has its roots in the legendary Shao Lin temple in Henan Province, China, said to have been founded in the fifth century, CE, by the Buddhist monk, Bodhidharma. According to legend, Bodhidharma came from India (though some accounts say he may have been Persian) to visit the Buddhist monks and assist them in their spiritual cultivation. Finding the monks in poor health due to physical inactivity, it was said that he introduced many forms of physical training that eventually led to the creation of Shao Lin Gong Fu, making the monks famous for their martial skill even to the present day. One of these practices that it is said he gave the monks is the qigong known as Yi Jin Jing ("Tendon Changing Practice").

While it in some parts resembles yoga, the original form is a fairly rigorous set of twelve movements designed to strengthen muscles, tendons, and bones, promote flexibility, qi, and blood circulation, develop speed, stamina, balance, and coordination, and to condense qi within the joint spaces to prevent their injury during martial training and engagement. The practice requires a fusion of attention, will, and physical strength, resulting in physical power amplified by condensed qi, and a calm, tranquil mind through the discharging of negative qi and the balancing of existing positive qi.

The traditional form is fairly popular among martial artists and those wishing to prevent or address arthritic conditions and osteoporosis, or to rehabilitate joints. The external form was adapted by Tom Tam after he took a group to China to learn the traditional form from a Shao Lin monk in May of 1992, and is especially useful for those wishing to develop the internal martial power, jin, utilized in Tai Qi, Xin Yi, Ba Gua and Wu Dao. Nicknamed "Chinese weightlifting" by many of his students, it is a very helpful practice in maintaining a healthy structure.

Position One: wu qi

Many qigong styles begin with some variation of this posture. It is designed to calm the mind and initiate qi-flow before the movements begin.

Wu qi refers to the condition of the universe before it came into form. It is considered a state of pure potential energy, gathering, circulating in on itself and promoting a state of movement within stillness.

Stand loosely with your head upright, eyes and gaze relaxed. The tip of the tongue should rest lightly in the space between the teeth and roof

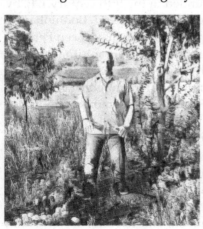

of the mouth; this connects the two central meridians, called the ren and du channels (also known as the "Conception Vessel" and "Governing Vessel", respectively), which feed the other meridian pathways and their organs. The knees are straight but not locked. All tension should be released, using only the muscle tension needed to hold oneself upright, but no more. Pay special attention to any tension that may be held in the stomach, chest, buttocks, and hips, and release it. The feet stand at shoulders' width, and the body is aligned so that the bone structure holds the majority of the weight of the body, allowing the muscles to relax further.

Open the hands lightly, softly round out the elbows (so that the approximate space of the width of one finger is apparent under the armpits), and hollow out the chest by rounding the shoulders forward, slightly.

Gently align the center of the palms over the tops of the feet. This connects three meridians: the pericardium, the liver, and the kidney channels. Breathing is slow, even, and silent. Bring attention to the Great Sea of Qi, the space located approximately one and a half cun (i.e. the length of the middle joint of the middle finger) below the navel and two-thirds of the way in towards the center of the abdomen.

At this point, there may be some heat, tingling, coolness or sensations of movement in the hands, feet, abdomen, and throughout the body. This is normal. This is the beginning of conscious qi circulation.

One may stay in this posture for as long as it feels right. In some traditions, the posture of wu qi is itself an entire qigong form, combined with a series of breathing and visualization exercises.

For the purposes of this form, most people hold this posture for three to five minutes, though it is perfectly acceptable to hold it for longer. Many hold the position for as long as thirty minutes in an effort to release stress and tension. (Two to three minutes in periods throughout the day often goes a long way towards making an otherwise stressful day more pleasant.)

Position Two: lengthen the spine, press the shoulders and fists down

Gently inhale, raise the hands to approximately the height of the lowest rib, and form two loose fists. On the exhale tighten the fists, lengthen the spine, slightly tuck the chin, pushing the top of the head up while simultaneously pressing the shoulders and fists down alongside the outsides of the legs.

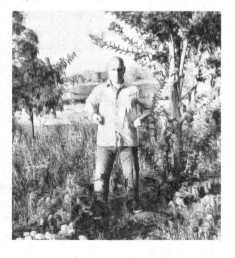

Breathing should be long, slow, and as free from tension as possible. Imagine that, on the inhale, the breath condenses in the abdominal cavity.

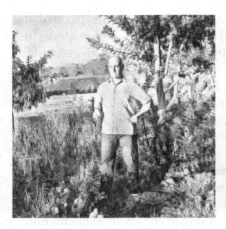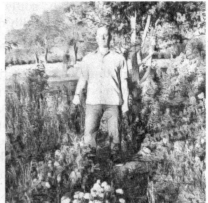

On the exhale, imagine that the breath flows through the arms and beyond the fists as well as through the soles of the feet and into the ground for approximately two meters. Hold the position for three to five seconds.

Once the exhale is complete, relax the fists and spine. Inhale, gently raising the loose fists to the lowest rib once again, and exhale, repeating the process anywhere from seven to forty-nine times, depending on what one's physical condition will allow.

This movement series develops "root"—the quality of qi density that sinks energy through and below the body. The action of pressing the shoulders down is the key to this flow. The positioning of the shoulders is one way to direct the flow of qi in the body. If the shoulders are raised, the qi rises. As they are dropped, the qi follows this action.

"Root" is considered important in qi development. The lower qi sits in the body, the less it is consumed unnecessarily, similar to how limiting the amount of airflow in a wood-burning stove will conserve fuel while providing ample heat. Sinking the qi is also useful in managing fear, anger, and mental confusion—all signs that the qi is sitting too high, putting stress on the heart and nervous system while depriving the immune system.

Position Three: extend and turn the arms and fists

Inhale to the abdominal cavity forming two loose fists in front of the chest with the elbows bent and pointing away from the sides of the body.

Exhale, lengthening the spine, tucking the chin, pushing up the top of the head while extending the arms at the height of the shoulders and tightening the fists.

Once the arms are lengthened fully, rotate the arms at the shoulders, turning the fists forward and down, so that the knuckle of each index finger is parallel with the ground, while at the same time trying

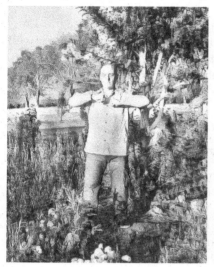 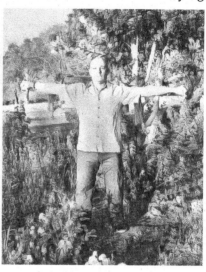

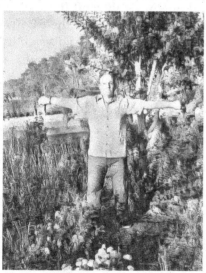

to extend the arms out farther, imagining that the exhale flows out through the fists, extending at least two meters beyond the width of the body in both directions, holding for three to five seconds.

This action opens the lung meridian and stimulates the nerves that activate the thymus gland, a key for strong immunity. It also conditions the wei qi, sometimes referred to as "guardian qi," the energy that surrounds the body, usually one to three meters in all directions. (Repeat from seven up to forty-nine times.)

Wei qi is considered the first line of defense in the body's immune system, responding to any substance or vibration that enters into one's qi field, alerting the body to begin its process of balancing, harmonizing or expulsion, depending ON what is appropriate. Well-conditioned wei qi is valuable in sensing and harmonizing with one's environment, as well as enabling one to sense the attention of others (because energy follows attention) as well as recognizing the intent behind that attention.

Martial artists cultivate dense and sensitive wei qi to sense the direction of an incoming attack before any movement takes place, as well as training their wei qi to respond to that flow of energy and absorb, redirect, or turn back its force. Highly skilled practitioners often cause opponents to stumble, temporarily freeze or lose coordination, with little or no apparent movement.

Position Four: point and lift the elbows

Inhale to the abdominal cavity while bending the elbows, pointing them forward, placing loose fists by the ears.

Exhale, pressing the fists down toward the shoulders while raising the elbows, imagining that the exhale flows through the elbows, forward from the body, about two meters, as the spine is lengthened, the chin, tucked, and the top of the head pushed skyward. As the elbows are raised and the fists pressed down, gently shift the weight back on the heels, setting the hips back at the same time the elbows are being lifted. Hold for three to five seconds. (Repeat from seven to forty-nine times.)

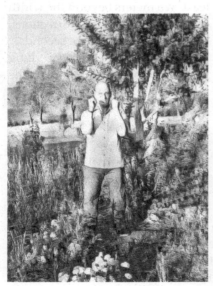 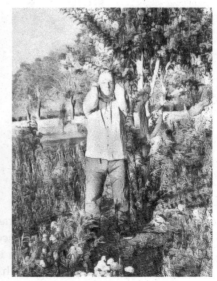

This action opens the mid back, improving qi-flow from the spine to the digestive organs, and relieves qi congestion around the heart, calming the mind and preventing inflammation around the heart. It is considered a good technique to discharge the effects of worry.

Position Five: extend the arms forward, turn the fists toward each other

Inhale to the abdomen, relaxing the fists at the sides of the body.

On the exhale, raise the arms, circling the fists past the sides of the ribcage (similar to a locomotive action), extending the arms forward at chest height, while the spine lengthens, the chin is tucked, and the top of the head pushes up.

Once the arms are fully extended, flex the wrists, turning the fists to face each other, imagining that the exhale extends through the lateral wrist creases, forward, beyond the body about two meters, being mindful not to lift the shoulders. As the arms extend, shift the weight back on the heels, setting the waist back. This will add an additional stretch to the tendons of the arms and hands, as the position is held for three to five seconds. (Repeat from seven to forty-nine times.)

This action helps develop and strengthen zhong qi, the energy that pervades the chest cavity, strengthening the lungs, heart, and thymus

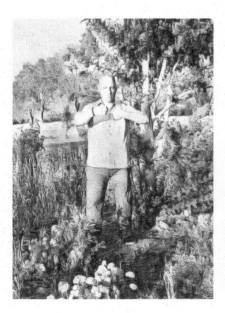
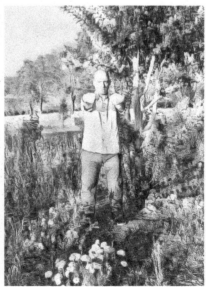

gland. It is also a way to discharge the energy of grief and sorrow; a way to reestablish the energy of joy that may have been compromised.

Martial artists use this exercise to augment striking power. The stretch of the tendons, exhaling imagery, and the flexing of the wrists all condense the qi in the fists and forearms. It is sometimes used in the series of exercises to develop "iron palm" skills and strength for qin na (seizing and locking an opponent's joints).

Position Six: press the palms, push forward the elbows

Inhale to the abdomen and raise the palms to face each other at about solar plexus height.

Exhale, pressing the palms with fingers together and pulled back. Bring the bent elbows forward so that the fingertips point to the hips. Imagine that the exhale flows through the palms.

At the same time as the palms press down, the head turns, first to the right side. Bring the palms together at the solar plexus on the inhale, and on the exhale press the palms down again and turn the head to the left, exhaling through the palms once more. Hold each position for three to five seconds. (Repeat from seven to forty-nine times.)

This series improves qi-flow through the spinal cord, improving the function of the central nervous system. At the same time, the

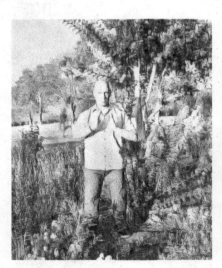
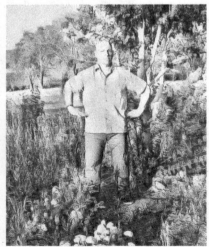

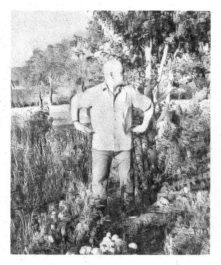

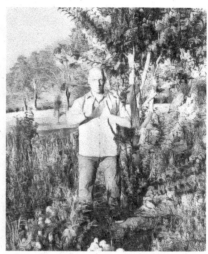

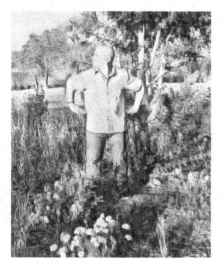

position of the elbows and the pressing of the palms harmonizes the pericardium meridian with the heart meridian, and dredges the gallbladder meridian of congestion. These movements further assist in calming the mind and can be helpful in relieving headaches and mental stress.

Martial artists use this to further augment "iron palm" techniques, especially the "falling tree" strikes that are common to some systems of Tai Qi.

Position Seven: turn in the feet, rotate the waist

Lower the fists to rest on the hips, with the elbows bent, extended to each side. Widen the stance to approximately one and a half times the width of the shoulders, and turn the feet slightly, in towards each other.

Inhale to the abdominal cavity.

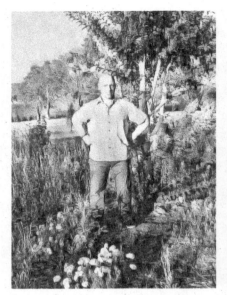

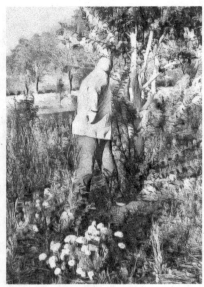

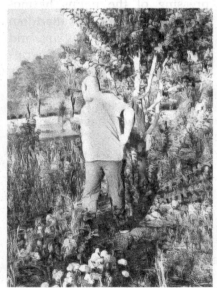

On the exhale, turn at the waist, first to the left, looking behind, gazing at the right heel, while imagining that the exhale flows down the backs of the legs, through the heels, about two meters into the ground.

Inhale into the abdominal cavity and return back to the center position.

Exhale down the backs of the legs, through the heels, two meters into the ground, turning right at the waist, looking behind at the left heel. Hold each side for three to five seconds. (Repeat, on each side, from seven to forty-nine times.)

These movements are designed to strengthen the qi of the kidneys and bladder, the water element, and to direct the qi deep inside the bone marrow, strengthening bones and nourishing blood. These actions also help to discharge the energy of anger and frustration, often stored in the liver and gallbladder, and to strengthen the energy of willpower, stored in the kidneys and bladder, and to improve brain function, influenced by the energy of bone marrow. It is also useful to help one regain vitality after a long illness or period of convalescence.

Position Eight: extend the heel across the center line

Maintaining the fists at rest on the hips, inhale the abdomen.

Exhale, raising a left bent knee to about waist height, then extending the heel across the right side of the center of the body, pulling the toes back and pushing the heel forward.

Imagine the breath flowing out the extended heel, holding the position for three to five seconds.

Inhale, bend the extended knee and place the foot back to its standing position.

Exhale, raise a bent right knee to about waist height, extend the heel across the body's center line to the left, pulling the toes back and pushing out the heel, imagining the breath flowing out through the extended heel, also for three to five seconds. (Repeat from seven to forty-nine times on each side.)

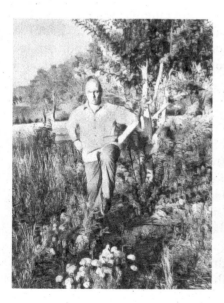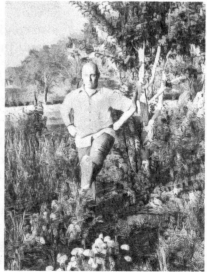

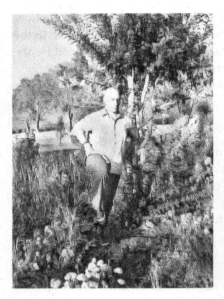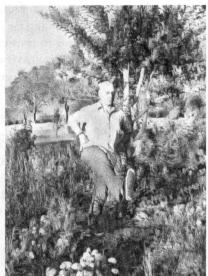

This exercise is designed to discharge the energy of fear and anxiety, often stored in the kidneys and bladder. Regular practice will improve balance, which also helps to improve cognitive function and mental stability.

Martial artists often use these movements to improve the strength of their stances, "root" balance, and the ability to adapt to changing conditions. It also condenses qi in the knees and feet, for improved kicking power, and protection against knee strikes and leg sweeps.

Position Nine: low "side blade" leg extension

Still keeping the fists at rest on the hips, inhale to the abdomen.

On the exhale, raise a left bent knee to approximately waist height, extend the leg laterally at about 45 degrees, rotating at the hip and piper thigh and flexing at the ankle, causing the foot to turn and push out the lateral side of the edge of the foot, similar to a completed "side blade" kick, at roughly a height between the knee and waist, while still maintaining an upright torso.

Imagine the exhale flows through the extended heel, while continuing to rotate at the hip and upper thigh, holding the position for three to five seconds.

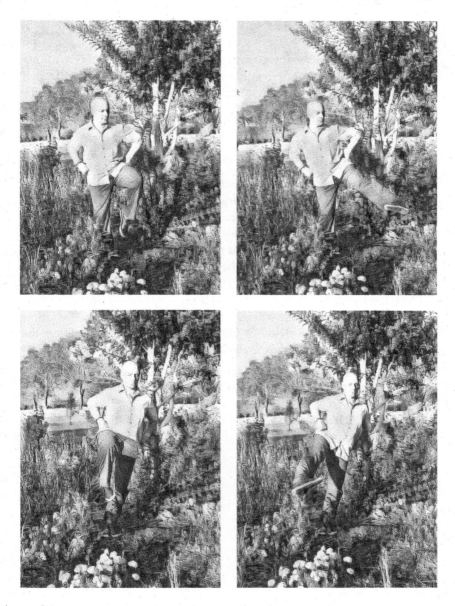

Inhale, return to the starting standing position, and follow the above steps with the right leg. (Repeat from seven to forty-nine times on each side.)

These actions are designed to strengthen the flow of qi though the gallbladder meridian, augmenting liver function, further discharging the stored energies of anger and frustration, and balancing the qi of the heart.

Martial artists will use these movements to stabilize the pelvis, allowing for qi to condense more deeply in the abdominal cavity, for stronger stances and balance, and an ability to maintain composure while under threat.

Position Ten: raise and lower the heels, circulate the qi

Bring the stance back to shoulders' width, and turn the heels out slightly. Place the hands, palms up, with fingertips almost touching, about six centimeters in front of the abdomen.

Inhale to the abdomen as the heels come off the ground and the body is balanced on the balls of the feet. At the same time, keeping the hands at the same width and distance from the body, raise the palms to the height of the solar plexus.

Once the inhale is complete, and the body is raised on the balls of the feet and the hands are at the height of the solar plexus, turn the palms over, keeping the same distance between the hands but bringing the palms close to the body by approximately three centimeters.

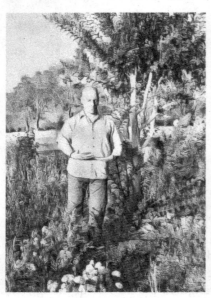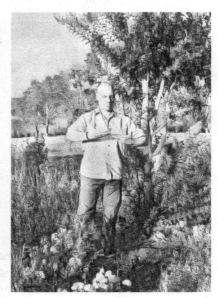

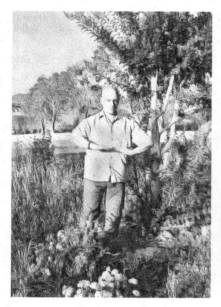 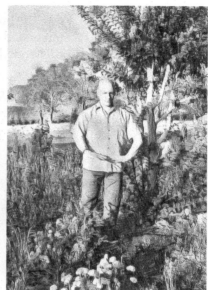

Exhale through the balls of the feet, about two meters into the ground, as the palms lower to the abdomen and the heels come to rest on the ground. The breathing and the movements should be slow and even. (Repeat from seven to forty-nine times.)

This action improves qi storage by drawing the qi still lower in the body through the action of raising and lowering the heels, and by raising and lowering the palms to circulate qi in the entire lower dantien.

Martial artists use these movements to unify the flow of qi and movement in the body so that the qi and physical body act as a single unit. This helps dissipate blows that land on the body, distributing the kinetic force throughout the whole structure and down through the root so that the strike will not "stick" in any one place. It also helps in unifying body, qi, and intent behind each technique.

Closing the form

Return to the opening wu qi position and breathe, using either the Buddhist or Daoist style breath, depending on the goal of training. For health purposes, Buddhist style breath is recommended. For martial purposes, Daoist. Make sure the breath is slow, even, and gentle, with little to no force. It is recommended to hold this position for three to five minutes, though it may be extended for meditative purposes for as long as one desires.

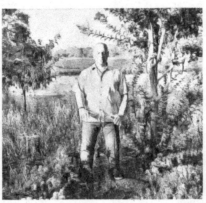

Moving neigong: Tai Qi Dao Yin practice

The form was created by Tom Tam to use the health-promoting aspects of Tai Qi but with simpler, less demanding movements. The intent of the exercise is to balance, store, and circulate qi for better health, a calm mind, and to improve one's sensitivity to qi.

Tai Qi Quan is one of the four traditional Chinese internal martial arts. Legend has it that it was created by Cheng, Sanfeng, a Daoist adept said to have achieved immortality. The story of his creating Tai Qi Quan says that he observed a bird attacking a snake. The snake remained still but alert as the bird maneuvered to attack, until, at the critical moment, the snake lunged forward with a fatal bite. He combined these observed techniques with his martial knowledge of White Crane and the health-promoting techniques of neigong, creating a sophisticated martial art that effectively defends the practitioner, should the need arise, while maintaining and improving his or her health.

The legend further states that, after applying his extensive knowledge of martial and healing techniques, he dreamt of a detailed sequence of movements he called "the long river," which combined all of his knowledge in a such a way as to be most beneficial to the practitioner. He awoke, it was said, with a sense of incredible qi power surging through his body.

101

While some claim to know the original sequence of movements that Sanfeng taught to his early disciples, most agree that the original sequence was lost over time. Few can even agree as to the number of movements in his routine.

One way *dao yin* may be translated is as "sensing the flow of natural energy." It was an early name for what was later termed "qigong." The "Tai Qi" in the name Tai Qi Dao Yin refers to the principles or method used to achieve the dao yin experience.

Position One: wu qi

The form opens with wu qi. (See above, p. 86)

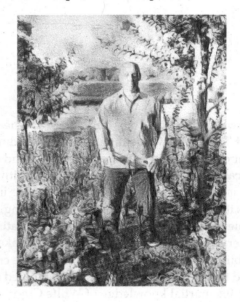

Position Two: gathering qi from heaven and earth

From wu qi, gently turn over the hands so that the palms are facing up. Keep the hands relaxed, using only enough strength to open them. Keeping a slight bend in the elbows, and, with shoulders relaxed, slowly raise the palms to the height of the armpit creases. Turn the hands over, gently, so that the palms face downwards, lowering them, holding your hands open and relaxed, back to the wu qi position. Repeat these movements from six to thirty-six times.

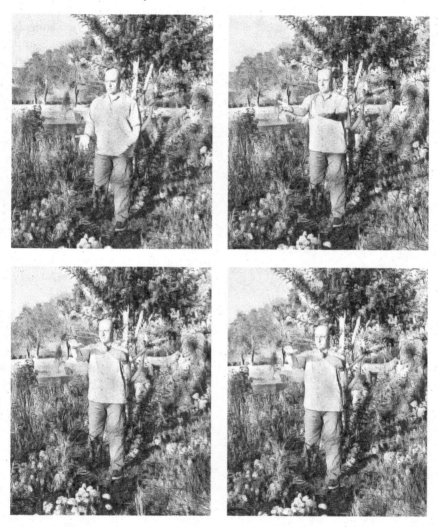

The movement is performed as if one were submerged in water. The time taken to raise the hands is the same as lowering them. Movements come from the shoulder, letting the larger joints move the smaller ones. It is sometimes helpful to imagine that the bend in the elbow is weighted; this may add to qi sensations.

This movement is designed to gather the surrounding qi (classically referred to as celestial qi and earthly qi) into the body through

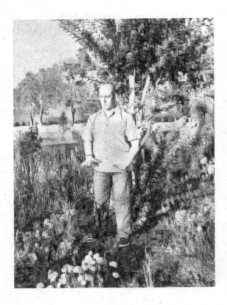

hands and arms, where the three upper body yin meridians, pericardium, heart, and lung, traverse. The very center of the palm, designated as Pericardium 8, "The Palace of Weariness" (Lao Kung), is a hugely influential point for absorbing and conducting qi.

The less tension in the body, the more qi can be conducted and absorbed. This second action of the form is designed to "fuel" the rest of the dao yin form, energizing the hands to conduct and balance the qi that is absorbed. Keep the movements slow, even, steady and, of course, relaxed.

Position Three: leading the qi from Yin Tang to the dantien

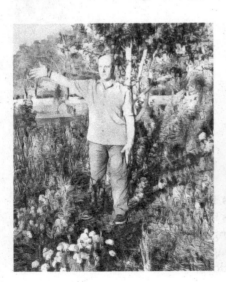
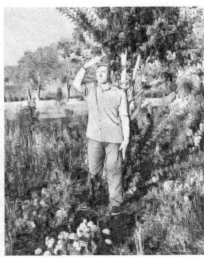

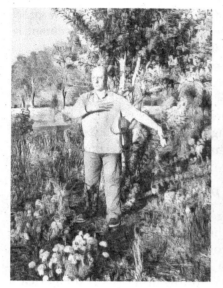

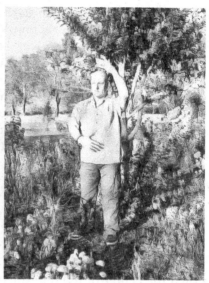

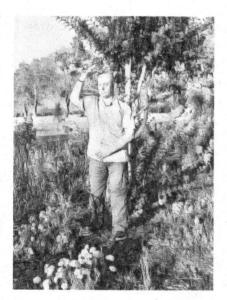

Upon completion of the previous movement, one is in wu qi position. Slowly raise the right hand up in line with the shoulder, circling the palm so that the center faces the center point between the eyebrows, approximately six to eight centimeters away from the body.

Slowly trace a line with the palm down the center line of the front of the body to the area designated as the lower dantien, just below the navel. As one palm completes the line, the next palm begins, and traces its line from the point between the eyebrows down to the point below the navel. There should be a slow, gentle, and continuous flow to these movements. Let the completion of first the right then the left hand be equal to one repetition. Repeat these movements from six to thirty-six times.

This portion of the form is designed to stimulate the flow of qi through the ren or "Conception Vessel" meridian. This movement is designed to store qi in the lower dantien.

The point between the eyebrows is called Yin Tang, referred to as "The Hall of the Spirit" or the "third eye." It is considered as the point that assists the energetic functions of the intellectual, intuitive, and spiritual aspects of the mind, where the aspects meet and blend in a harmonious interplay. It is also thought of as a bridge between the brain (intelligence, logic) and the heart (intuition, spiritual connection).

Position Four: leading the qi to the palace

Extend the left arm, palm facing up, relaxed and with a moderate bend in the elbow, at about the height of your chest. Bringing the right palm to the center of your chest, still approximately six to eight centimeters away, trace a line from the center of the chest down the center of the interior part of the arm (this is the pericardium meridian), down to the left palm and extending beyond your fingertips. While tracing with the right palm, the left arm draws back until the right palm has passed the left fingertips.

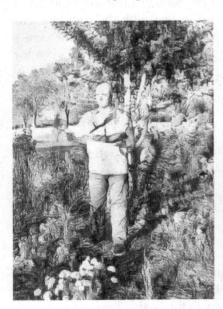
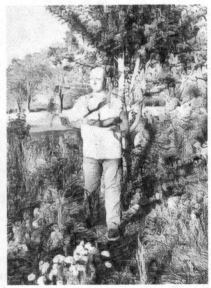

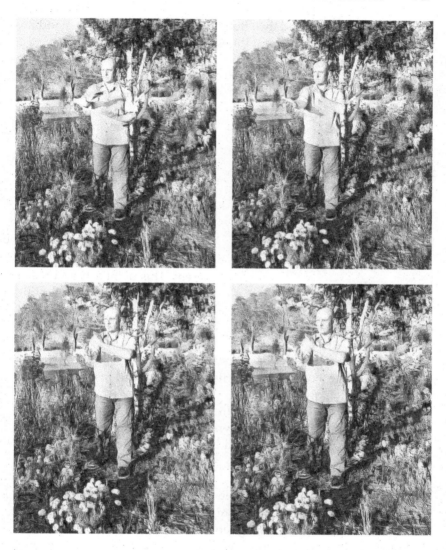

With the right arm now extended in front of the chest, turn it over so that the palm faces up. At the same time, turn over the left palm, bring it to face the center of the chest, then trace a line down the center of the right arm; the right arm draws back until the left palm passes the center of the palm and fingertips. As always, the key to this movement is keeping the tension out of the hands and arms. Leading the qi first through the left pericardium meridian, and then through the right pericardium meridian, counts as one repetition. Repeat this six to thirty-six times.

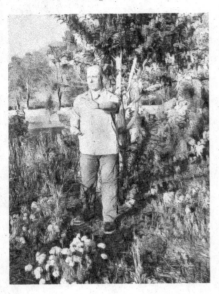

The purpose of this part of the form is to stimulate qi-flow to all of the upper body yin meridians (pericardium, heart, and lung) and bring them into harmony with each other. The center of the palm, in the line between the ring and middle fingers is designated as the acupuncture point, Pericardium 8, also known as "The Palace of Weariness" (Lao Gong) for its restorative functions, particularly when there is exhaustion present. This point acts as a major channel of qi, both in collecting and emitting; that is, it may draw in qi in order to strengthen, or it may emit qi in order to assist the balance and healing of another person through the use of Fa Gong as a means of therapy. For this reason, its magnetic functions make it very useful in directing qi movement.

Pericardium 5, the acupuncture point located approximately a quarter of the way between the wrist and elbow crease, is the point where the pericardium, heart, and lung meridians converge, making the pericardium meridian ideal to promote qi circulation throughout the body.

With this movement most people who have just begun their qigong practice often experience the most qi. It is common to experience a sensation of warmth, tingling, a magnetic sensation, a cooling sensation, or any combination of these. However, one ought not to be too concerned if there isn't a sensation of qi right away, or if it seems strong one day and subtle the next. All of this reflects a state of body both internally and externally. Sensations may even vary in type and intensity at different times of day. As practice and cultivation of qi grow, the qi sensations experienced first in the hands will likely be experienced throughout the whole body.

Position Five: Master Yan Xin's posture

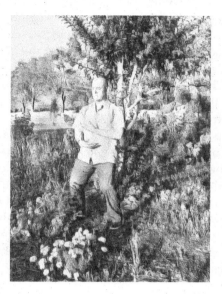

Place the right hand, palm turned up, approximately three centimeters below the navel. Place the left hand, palm turned up, at the level of the solar plexus and directly over the right hand, so that the palms are in line with each other. Both hands are about six centimeters away from the body. Step out with either the right or left foot, so that the distance between the feet is approximately a shoulders' width plus one half. Bend both knees, slightly tucking the pelvis, as if sitting on a very high stool. Position the solar plexus forward slightly, and gently tuck your chin as if glancing down. As always, remember to keep the torso and hands as free from tension as possible. Hold this position anywhere from one to five minutes.

This posture is adapted from a qigong system designed by Master Yan Xin. By itself, the posture is a very effective method of cultivation, as is Master Yan's Nine Step qigong system. For the purposes of this form, this movement was adapted to regulate the "three burning spaces" in the body.

The triple heater meridian, the yang compliment to the pericardium meridian, is considered the body's "consummate host." It harmonizes the organs in the lower, middle, and upper spaces (designated as the lower abdomen, upper abdomen, and thoracic regions, respectively). This posture also has the effect of regulating the endocrine system, and is particularly useful in nourishing the adrenal glands.

The bent-knee stance is called *ma bu* or "Horse Stance". It is designed to activate the "root" of the body's qi, bringing the qi through the legs, feet, and into the ground.

The legs, in Chinese medicine, are considered to be the "second heart," meaning that one of the keys to having a strong and healthy heart is to have strong legs.

Tucking your pelvis and chin and bringing the solar plexus forward have the effect of opening the "three gates" of the spinal cord: C7, where the neck meets the shoulders; T12, where the thoracic spine meets the lumbar spine; and L5, where the lumbar spine meets the sacrum. It also gently opens the point between the second and third lumbar vertebra, called "The Gate of Destiny." The position also has the effect of opening the spine. The spine, in Chinese medicine, is called the "Heavenly Pillar," the main conductor of celestial qi, and is the physical location of the Governing Vessel.

Position Six: storing the qi in the dantien

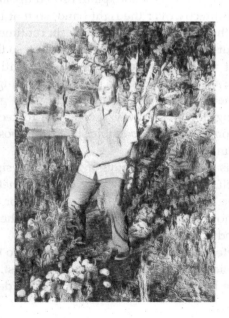

Remaining in the position of Master Yan Xin's posture, place a palm about one and a half cun below your navel on your abdomen. Place the other palm on top of the first hand, so that the centers of both palms line up with the point one and a half cun below the navel. Hold this position anywhere from one to five minutes.

This posture is meant to store and condense the qi in the dantien. The point one and a half cun below the navel is designated as Conception Vessel 6, or "The Great Sea of Qi." As was said earlier, this point is one gateway to a reservoir of qi. This posture is designed to bring the circulation of qi into the dantien, "charging the battery," and, over time, increasing a body's ability to store qi. As qi is circulated throughout the abdomen, the body's alarm (*mu*) points are stimulated. The alarm points could be likened to the organs' "circuit breakers." They are especially useful in acupuncture treatment if there are any organs in distress. Coupling these movements with the straight spine position makes for a very balanced, powerful, and efficient exercise.

Position Seven: Iron Shirt

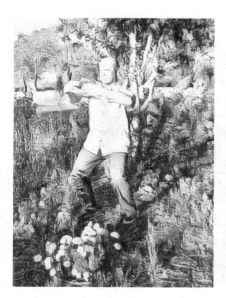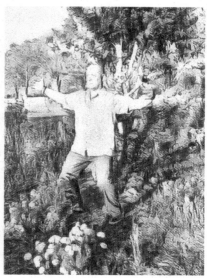

Staying in the same stance as the previous two positions, and keeping shoulders, arms, and hands relaxed, extend the arms in front, so that the palms are facing the chest, at about the height of the crease of the armpits. Fingertips should be lined up with each other, and elbows are

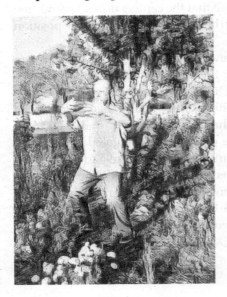

loose and hanging, as if weighted. Allow the hands to drift apart to about the width plus one half of the body, and then allow them to drift back to being directly in front of the chest. Typically, though not always, the arms expand outward at the pace of one inhalation, and come back to the front of the chest at the pace of one exhalation. Repeat this movement from six to thirty-six times.

The Iron Shirt posture is taken from a series of martial arts qigong exercises designed to condition the body to be less vulnerable to injury when attacked.

For the purposes of this form, the posture is used to balance the concentration of qi in the meridians on the left and right sides of the body.

Known as an *akabani* imbalance in some systems of acupuncture, an imbalance of qi on either side of the body often leads to one-sided symptoms in the body. (A person with fibromyalgia, for example, will often experience more pain on one side of the body than another.)

The posture also strengthens a protective field of qi around the body (wei qi). The field is considered a first line of defense in illness, and also helps one to remain more energetically self-contained, preventing unwanted influence from negative sources, either from the immediate environment or the dispositions of others.

Position Eight: extend qi to the limbs

Returning to the original wu qi position, cross the hands, palms facing the chest, about eight centimeters in front. Separate the hands, gently pushing palms out to either side of the body and extending the left leg to the side of the body while balancing on the right leg. Then cross hands again in the same manner, press out palms, and extend the right leg while balancing on the left leg. Repeat this movement three to six times on each side.

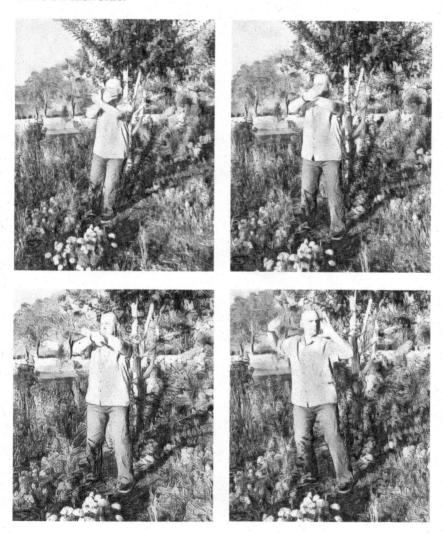

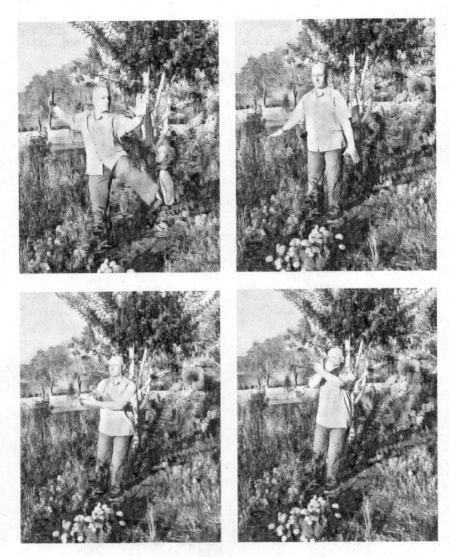

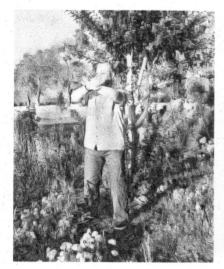
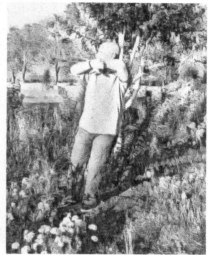

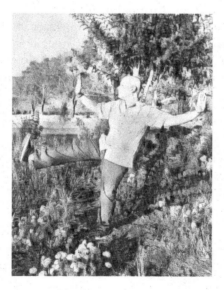

This portion of the form is used to integrate the movement of qi that has taken place throughout the rest of the exercises. As an exercise in balance, it has the effect of stimulating the motor cortex of the brain. (Most exercises in Chinese medicine designed to prevent senility have many balancing postures to help activate and harmonize brain centers.)

Position Nine: condensing the qi in the dantien, *and closing the forms*

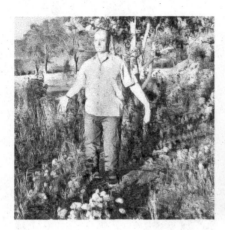
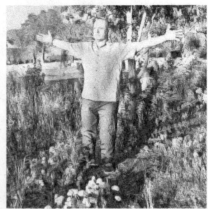

Return to wu qi position. Turn palms up, raise the arms at your sides, then circle the hands around so that the palms face your forehead. Softly "press" the palms down in front, as if gently packing and condensing qi into the abdomen. When the palms reach the abdomen, turn them out again, circling up again, repeating this movement six to thirty-six times.

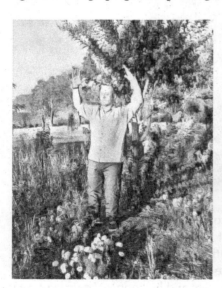
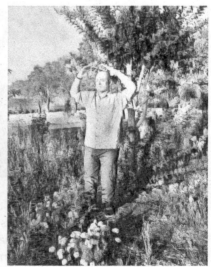

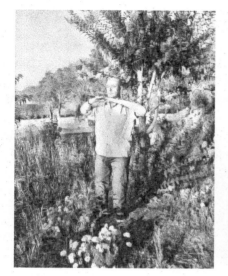

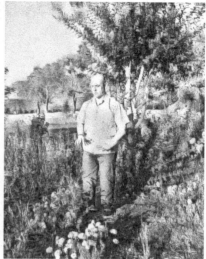

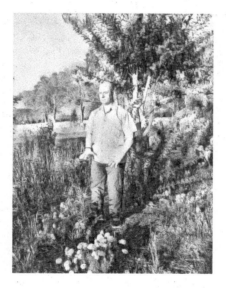

This final portion of the form serves as its closing. Qi has been moved throughout the body, achieving relative balance. The increased qi-flow is returned to the body's "storage tank," the dantien. The dantien allows a body to store and condense qi without limit.

Neigong: Zhan Zhuang
Cheng Bao ("Tree Hugging")

The term "Zhan Zhuang" may be translated, literally, as "standing like a post." To an outward observer, little appears to be happening—short of someone standing very still in a static posture. For the practitioner, there is a great deal of activity. Zhan Zhuang postures initiate a great deal of qi movement and, over time, are excellent means of qi cultivation and development.

Originally a Daoist health practice, Zhan Zhuang gained a great deal of popularity when Wang Xiangzhai developed a method of internal martial arts based on Xin Yi Quan called *Yi Quan* ("Intent Fist"). (It is said that he coined the term "standing like a post" to describe the fundamental stages of training.) The martial goal is to develop a strong fusion of qi and body structure, making the postures popular among most internal stylists. For health benefits, it is an excellent method for clearing obstructed qi-flow in the body, calming the central nervous system, and healing muscular-skeletal conditions.

The main principles of Zhan Zhuang emphasize training yi (consciousness, intent), proper body alignment, and a harmonious relaxation of body and mind, resulting in the mastery of xing (form), yi (intent), li (strength), *qi* (energy), and shen (mental and spiritual presence). As a health-promoting practice, the postures stimulate cardiovascular activity, neuromuscular coordination, and efficient metabolism. Their benefits have been studied in the treatment of arthritis, neurasthenia, hypertension, and gastrointestinal and respiratory disorders, and have reportedly been useful as part of a treatment strategy for post-traumatic stress.

Yi (intent) is the basis of this system. The stances are designed to enhance the efficient transfer of qi, circulating it through the organs and medians, gradually condensing it in the body's cavities, joint spaces, and tendons. The mind's intent is used to amplify the effects of the posture and eventually will play a leading role through imagery, breath control, and leading the qi to the dantien (lower abdominal cavity), "root" (through the feet and deep into the ground), and extended through the limbs and gradually in all directions like an inflating ball.

Spiritually, the stances aid in mastering one's primal tendencies. A deep stance will eventually become painful. The impulses to rise out of it, to shift out of proper alignment or to give in to frustration will all present themselves. Training one's will to remain calm and still strengthens one's consciousness in subduing impulses, helping the practitioner gain mastery of him or herself.

Practitioners often report a sense of interconnectedness both internally and externally. Many people practice Zhan Zhuang Qigong exclusively, achieving outstanding results in health, wellbeing, and skill.

Cheng Bao Zhuang ("Tree Hugging Stance")

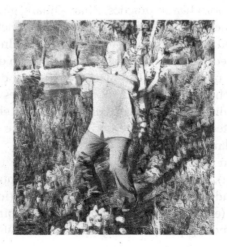

The stance is, by far, the most popular, utilized by those seeking both good health and martial ability. Many practitioners of neigong and, in particular, Zhan Zhuang, use only this posture as their complete practice.

There are many variations to this posture, particularly with regards to the angle and shape of the hands. While many practitioners regard a different execution of the posture than what they are used to as "wrong," that conclusion itself is likely to be erroneous. Most of the variations produce good results in health and martial ability. Hands, feet, arms, legs, ears, and scalp are all seen, in qigong and Chinese medical theory, as miniature representations of the whole body, as holographic models that influence the entire body. (For example, the shape of the ear may be likened to an upside-down fetus. The auricular acupuncture points target the corresponding parts of the body of that shape to affect the rest of the body.) Changing the shape of the hands subtly changes the way the qi is conditioned within the body's cavities and joints. As long as the spine, pelvis, and arms are properly aligned, with the legs bent at the proper angle and the body relatively free from tension, the qi will circulate and health and martial benefits will accumulate.

Feet: To begin, one stands with the feet at approximately shoulders' width.

Knees: The knees are bent, dropping the torso lower, the length of the distance of one hand, measured from the wrist crease to the top of the middle finger. As one's strength and stamina grow, one may lower to the length of two hands, to three, and so on, as long as the rest of the alignment remains in integrity.

Pelvis: The pelvis is slightly tucked under and forward, gently opening the space between the second and third lumbar vertebra, creating a sensation of the coccyx "hanging" while pointing towards the ground. It is important not to flex into this position, but, rather, to tilt the pelvis with as little tension as proper alignment will allow. Relax the waist as much as possible.

Spine: The spine should be held straight, upright, not leaning to either side.

Chest: The chest remains upright, but slightly hollowed. It should be relaxed enough to create a sensation of a slight cavity in the front of the chest, but not so much that the back bows, creating roundness in the upper back.

Head: Gently lift the top of the head by extending the neck and tucking the chin, lowering it approximately one cun.

Arms: Raise the arms with the elbows bent. The elbows are lower than the hands. The distance of the hands is two hand lengths (measured from the wrist crease to the tip of the middle finger) away from the chest. The wrists and hands are positioned at the height of the clavicle. The height of the tips of the elbows are just below the lower part of the crease of the armpits.

Hands: The hands are positioned as if they are loosely holding a bowl in front of the chest. The distance between them may range from one half to twice the width of one hand. The fingertips of the left and right hands point toward each other.

Breathing: Inhale slowly and evenly. The intention initially brings the breath to the lower dantien (one and a half cun below the navel). On the exhale, the intention directs the breath through the soles of the feet, roughly one to two meters into the ground.

Eyes: The eyes are half closed and hold a soft gaze between the hands.

Imagery and sensation: When one first begins post standing training, one may find it somewhat challenging, but as strength, calm, and stamina grow, the results quickly become apparent.

An often overlooked training component is using one's intention to harmonize with the force of gravity. The practitioner notices the places where the body feels especially "weighted" (very often these are the bends in the arms, the shoulders, and the hands) and puts attention on that feeling as if to add even more density to the sensation. As this is happening, the waist, abdomen, shoulders, hips, and buttocks are consciously relaxed, so that most of the pressure felt in keeping the integrity of the posture is felt in the quadriceps. All this continues while maintaining a "plumb line" from the top of the head (located by measuring two lines from the tops of the ears to the top of the skull) through the center of the body, beyond the pelvic floor, and straight through, one to two meters into the ground.

Even conditioned athletes are often surprised at how much their legs and shoulders ache with fatigue after a short time. Some beginners notice a sharp increase in heartbeat, profuse sweating, shaking, and a desire to sway. (It is best to hold still in the posture, despite the desire to sway. If that isn't possible, one may find it best to end the training session, even if it has only lasted a short time.) Others may experience emotional agitation with strong feelings of anger, anxiety or sadness.

This is all normal.

The position creates an environment in the body where qi may flow, balance and accumulate, fusing with the structure and discharging disharmonious energies. The legs and shoulders may ache more as the qi and the structure fuse together. The heart rate may increase along with perspiration as a means of releasing old illness and emotions. Shaking and a desire to sway may happen as the qi breaks through obstructions to its flow. Old emotional disturbances and memories may surface and release through tears, sighing or groaning as their energetic charge is dissipated.

After a short period of daily training, typically ten to fourteen days, the posture becomes much more comfortable. The legs are strong enough that one feels as if one is "sitting" in the posture, allowing for further relaxation around the waist and torso, further increasing the downward flow of qi, building "root." The arms may feel buoyant, as if they are lightly floating on top of warm water, while the magnetic sensation of a large ball of qi expands around the arms and chest with each breath.

Many practitioners add the image of themselves as a tree with roots penetrating deep into the ground. The torso is a thick, powerful trunk; the arms and hands are strong branches.

Within a short time after the posture becomes easier, the ball of qi felt around the chest and arms will expand through the body in all directions, and then well beyond the body. At this point, the more tranquil one's mindset, the more one will sense and feel the qi as it extends beyond the body, connecting with the combined flow of qi from heaven and earth. At this stage, one's enhanced abilities begin to develop. One may develop the increased power that comes from qi fusing with and condensing within the physical body. One may sense the attention and intentions of those nearby. One may feel the communication of other living beings such as plants, animals, mountains, streams, or the Earth as a whole. For some, these abilities enter the realm of what is commonly called psychic ability. All of these enhanced abilities are inborn characteristics of human beings. They only require an increase in the volume of qi and the improving characteristics of virtue to elevate their functions.

Practice time: In the early stages it is not uncommon to find that one may not hold the posture longer than three to five minutes. As strength and patience increase, twenty to thirty minutes each day is considered optimal for health benefits. Many advanced martial artists will practice for one to two hours each day.

Additional thoughts on practice

Patience and persistence are invaluable. This often requires faith in the beginning, where one hasn't yet experienced the many beneficial effects of practice. Traditionally, it was said that the first one hundred days are critical to building a good foundation. This is also true for many activities that could benefit one's health, such as a new diet or exercise routine.

Metabolically, many of a body's cells are regenerated within that period, though some take longer, with red blood cells regenerating about every four months, and liver cells approximately every five months. If one maintains good discipline in qi cultivation, the newer cells are produced within a higher qi environment, creating potentially healthier cells and structures.

Proper form and mindset are essential. It is best to master a few movements or postures before moving on to the next. More benefit is gained through proper execution of one technique than improper execution of several. A popular saying among practitioners: "It is better to have one sharp knife than ten dull knives."

Grasp for nothing, yet welcome everything. Many people's desire for special abilities is often a hindrance to progress. This approach is sometimes referred to as having a "tight" mind, that is, a mind so fixated that it may not recognize other benefits or, being so restrictive, will not allow a full flow of qi, insisting on a particular stream instead. Some practitioners may hope to acquire clairvoyant ability, for example, when a true gift of being able to help others heal is one of their latent abilities.

Whatever benefits come to the surface, they are valuable steps to one's personal evolution and will streamline the process if they are embraced.

Enjoy the process. The development of qi and virtue offer fascinating and enriching experiences. The gifts of self-knowledge, confidence, calm, peace, intuition, and feelings of interconnectedness continuously unfold. It is as Lao Zi states in the *Dao De Ching*: "Without going outside, you may know the whole world."